The Mind-Body Interface in Somatization

The Mind-Body Interface in Somatization

When Symptom Becomes Disease

W. Lynn Smith, PhD
with Patrick W. Conway, MDiv,
and Jonathan O. Cole, MD

JASON ARONSON
Lanham • Boulder • New York • Toronto • Plymouth, UK

Published by Jason Aronson
An imprint of Rowman & Littlefield Publishers, Inc.
A wholly owned subsidiary of The Rowman & Littlefield Publishing Group, Inc.
4501 Forbes Boulevard, Suite 200, Lanham, Maryland 20706
http://www.rowmanlittlefield.com

Estover Road, Plymouth PL6 7PY, United Kingdom

British Library Cataloguing in Publication Information Available

Library of Congress Cataloging-in-Publication Data

Smith, W. Lynn (Wallace Lynn), 1922-
The mind-body interface in somatization : when symptom becomes disease / W. Lynn Smith ; with Patrick W. Conway and Jonathan O. Cole.
p. ; cm.
Includes bibliographical references and index.
ISBN 978-0-7657-0749-9 (cloth : alk. paper)
1. Somatization disorder. 2. Cognitive therapy. 3. Dialectical behavior therapy. I. Conway, Patrick W., 1951- II. Cole, Jonathan O. III. Title.
[DNLM: 1. Somatoform Disorders—etiology. 2. Mind-Body Relations (Metaphysics) 3. Mind-Body Therapies—methods. 4. Somatoform Disorders—therapy. WM 170 S663m 2010]
RC552.S66S65 2010
616.85'24—dc22 2009038952

∞™ The paper used in this publication meets the minimum requirements of American National Standard for Information Sciences—Permanence of Paper for Printed Library Materials, ANSI/NISO Z39.48-1992. Printed in the United States of America

This book is dedicated to the memory and life's work of my husband, Dr. Lynn Smith, who devoted fifty years of his life to research to find ways to help people, make their lives easier, and help them cope with their pain. Many of the chapters address the mind-body interaction involving the pain state. It is the authors' belief that a better understanding of the organic, physiological, and psychological correlation of pain will result in a more global understanding and more successful treatment of pain and the patient who suffers from it.

His loving wife,

Ria Smith

Contents

Preface

Somatization has been my fascination for over forty years. Early in my career as a practicing neuropsychologist, I was perplexed by the persistent post-surgical symptom complaints of patients who were, quite honestly, expected to respond favorably to treatment. Later, through my Cortical Function Laboratories at Porter Adventist Hospital in Denver and White Memorial Hospital in Los Angeles, I performed neuropsychological evaluations on an average of four hundred patients a year from nearly every medical specialty to assist in establishing differential diagnoses. Time and again, I listened to stories of ongoing pain-related disability and frustration as patients went from physician to physician in search of an elusive cure. Out of these experiences came my first journal publication, "Personality and the Relief of Chronic Pain: Predicting Surgical Outcome."[1]

In the course of psychotherapy with many more patients, I realized there was considerable underlying pathology at work which not only inhibited their response to medical treatment, but also seemed almost integral to their character structure. The more I probed into the meaning of their symptoms, the more resistant they became and the more frequently they withdrew from therapy. At the same time, I worked with other highly functional patients who were "stopped dead in their tracks" by illness or surgery. These individuals had no history of debilitation but were still unable to overcome the immediate effects of their condition. I gradually realized these patients were situationally affected and I came to believe there was genuine hope for a positive outcome if only the right treatment could be found. Both groups of patients suffered from somatization but there was a critical difference between them: For those in the former group, somatization seemed to be a way of life while those in the latter had been caught in midstride, so to speak, by a crisis they could not overcome. As a result, I began to think of somatization in terms of a chronic type and a situational type. Over the years, these experiences coalesced in the development of two objective testing instruments; that is, the Paindex® test and SDA® Screen (Somatic Displacement Analysis), which have proved invaluable in predicting the somatization response.

In the summer of 2000, I happened to be in the medical library of Porter Adventist Hospital in Denver, Colorado, where I met my coauthor, Patrick W. Conway, MDiv. By happy coincidence, we were both searching for information on personality theory and began to chat. As these things sometimes go, our brief conversation extended into several hours and a solid friendship was born. At the time I was planning a book detailing my experiences evaluating patients for the presence of somatization that I could use as a text with medical and psychiatric residents. Conway's experiences in pastoral counseling and psychotherapy with psychiatric patients dovetailed with my own in many aspects. Furthermore, we were both stymied by the fact that the professional literature failed to answer so many of the questions we were asking about somatization. Eventually we realized if a book was going to be written that addressed our concerns, we would have be the ones to write it. It is my sincere hope that clinicians and researchers will find our book as useful as we have found it rewarding.

W. Lynn Smith, PhD

NOTE TO THE READER

One always hopes a book will outlive its author. Life has a way of intervening unexpectedly, however, and that is certainly the case here. In the months immediately preceding the publication of this manuscript, W. Lynn Smith, PhD, and Jonathan O. Cole, MD, fell ill and passed away. I have been privileged to call both these men not only colleague and teacher, but also cherished friends.

The very existence of this book is due, first and last, to Dr. Smith's genius and determination. His experience in the field of neuropsychology and the diagnosis of somatizing syndromes provided not only its theoretical foundation, but also was the guiding principle throughout the research and preparation of the manuscript. His drive, energy, and sense of humor were an inspiration throughout many long hours of writing and editing. Although

---

Paindex® and SDA® screen are registered servicemarks, patented with the U.S. Department of Patents and Registration (Patent number US7, 097, 617 B1).

his honored career includes university professorships (University of North Dakota, University of Denver), research, and authorship, he was at his best in the clinical setting. Colleagues have described him as "the clinician's clinician." His seminal insights into the relationship between somatization and personality are not only highly original, they also are imminently practical. Dr. Smith wished this book to not only stimulate further research but also to inform and educate the physician, psychologist, and student. It has been my deepest privilege to have benefited from his knowledge, skill, and wisdom, and I trust our readers will find themselves enriched as they work through the pages of this, his last and my first, book. It is his legacy and stands as a tribute to a treasured friendship. Were it not for him, I would not be writing these words. The manuscript, with the exception of Dr. Cole's chapter on psychopharmacology, was complete before his death and his fingerprints are evident on every page. If only he had lived to see them in print.

Dr. Cole was a pioneer in the field of modern psychiatry and psychopharmacology. While his knowledge of medications was encyclopedic, even more valuable have been his insights into patient care and the genuine, unaffected manner in which he approached both patients and colleagues. Although he is chiefly known for his contributions to drug treatment, he had a lively interest in psychosomatic medicine as his contribution to this work indicates. His collegiality, careful instruction, and humor have inspired several generations of psychiatric clinicians, including this writer. To say he will be sorely missed is scarcely adequate.

Patrick W. Conway, MDiv

Acknowledgments

We would like to acknowledge the support of colleagues at the University of Colorado Health Sciences Center, Porter Adventist Hospital of Denver, and York Hospital in York, Maine. In particular, we wish to thank E. Andrew Jonassen, MD, and Charles Hamlin, MD, both Associate Clinical Professors of Orthopedics at the University of Colorado Health Sciences Center. Dr. Jonassen's support and encouragement in the course of our writing has been invaluable and we are deeply grateful for his friendship and confidence in our undertaking. For many years, Dr. Hamlin has relied on the Paindex® test to aid his evaluation of patients for response to surgery for pain relief. His friendship and collegiality remain an ongoing inspiration. We want to thank Joshua P. Cole, MD, of York Hospital for confirming the usefulness of our ideas in clinical practice; "thank you" hardly seems adequate. We also wish to acknowledge the time and generous assistance of the library staff of Porter Adventist Hospital, especially Mr. Richard Maxwell, Ms. Ellen Graves, and Ms. Connie Baker. We truly appreciate all your fine work. Finally, we wish to express our heartfelt gratitude to our wives and families, including Mr. Thomas Hood, for their faith, patience, and devotion during the research and preparation of this manuscript. Without them, our work would never have seen the light of day.

On behalf of all my coauthors, I'd like to express my appreciation to editors Julie Kirsch and Karen Ackermann and their staff at Jason Aronson, not only for seeing the potential in a work of this sort, but for their invaluable assistance, guidance, and support during the entire publication process.

Additionally, a special word of thanks is due to the executors of the estates of W. Lynn Smith, PhD, and Jonathan O. Cole, MD, for their gracious assistance in approving the publication of this manuscript.

Introduction

Somatic displacement or somatization is one of the most prevalent and least understood problems facing health care delivery today. Somatizing syndromes account for one-fourth to one-third of primary care visits and consume a staggering 80 percent of available health care dollars. Somatization is encountered in nearly every medical specialty and each one seems to have its own characteristic expression:

Rheumatology – fibromyalgia
Internal Medicine – chronic fatigue syndrome
Gastroenterology – irritable bowel syndrome
Rehabilitation Medicine – closed head injury
Endocrinology – multiple chemical sensitivity, hypoglycemia
Orthopedics – low back pain
Obstetrics/Gynecology – pelvic pain, premenstrual syndrome
Otolaryngology – tinnitus
Neurology – dizziness, headache
Cardiology – atypical chest pain
Pulmonary – hyperventilation, dyspnea
Dentistry – temperomandibular joint syndrome[1]

There is evidence to suggest that physician frustration with problematic patients is largely due to somatization and increased utilization of medical services.[2] Repeated and elaborate workups, medical specialty consultations, and treatments reflecting diagnostic uncertainty drain health care resources. In general practice, somatization is most typically regarded as a diagnosis of exclusion used only when other possibilities have been ruled out, resulting in somatization being underdiagnosed and undertreated.[3] There are legitimate reasons for this: a general practitioner (GP) may be unfamiliar with the terminology of somatization, s/he may not wish to attribute illness complaints to somatization simply because of a lack of diagnostic certainty, and there is the ethical desire to do something to help the patient even if it means providing only symptomatic treatment. Complicating this picture is the tendency of medical training to artificially divide health care into physiological and psychological aspects. Mind and body, however, do not submit so easily to these distinctions but clinicians may experience serious ambivalence about mind-body interactions and their role in effective health care delivery.

It has been said that we diagnose those disorders for which we have available treatments. In the case of somatization, treatment may be as ambiguous as diagnosis. We need to widen our perspective in order to understand how somatization produces identifiable physiologic dysfunction that defies typical medical classification. Doing so involves learning how somatization functions as a disease process that stems from the mind-body interface. We need to become more comfortable diagnosing somatization not only as a psychiatric comorbidity but also as the underlying process in the patient's clinical presentation. In order to do that, we need to know where somatization comes from and what factors contribute to its development.

In this volume, we offer a new perspective on the etiology of somatization that includes interpersonal, intrapersonal, and existential elements. Even a brief search of the current literature indicates a certain preoccupation with diagnosis based on the Diagnostic and Statistical Manual of Mental Disorders (DSM). To a certain extent this is understandable and even to be expected. As we discuss in detail in chapter 1, the DSM provides a clinically applicable, standardized set of diagnostic criteria. The problem is, however, that a great deal of the literature seems to concentrate on the elucidation of DSM categories to the exclusion of much else. Scientific description has displaced dynamic explanation, and we find this troubling. Ironically, even when a diagnosis has been determined, this is no guarantee that a healthy and productive doctor-patient relationship will be established.

We wish to transcend conventional thinking and answer the questions that have kept us up late at night: why do some patients somatize in the first place, is somatization a process or a diagnosis, can we predict who will somatize and who will not, why are these patients frequently treatment resistant, and can this condition even be treated effectively? We have written for the psychiatrist, psychologist, and medical clinician eager for new insights into the underlying dynamics and management of somatization. Masters level clinicians, nurses, and social workers will also find our volume useful because they are involved in the day-to-day care of these patients, especially in hospital settings. Specifically, the reader should anticipate meeting the following goals:

- Develop a more nuanced understanding of the etiology of somatization and its presentation
- Become more acquainted with the basis for conceptualizing the interface between mind and body
- Understand how ambivalence and progressive function in the two main subtypes of somatization
- Understand the role played by shame in the development of somatization
- Understand the ways in which personality can be predictive of somatization
- Become familiar with the basic tenants of psychotherapy for both subtypes
- Develop a greater appreciation for the complexities of using pharmacological interventions in somatization
- Gain a much greater sense of empathy for patients

If we understand that illness results from the combination of a vulnerable individual with a disease process (individual + disease = illness), we can see how somatization explains somatic syndromes and how treatment that neglects somatization is doomed to frustration. Somatic syndromes are the target of symptomatic treatment but the proclivity to somatization represents the underlying disease process. While the patient may experience some measure of symptomatic relief, the disease itself remains in place only to resurface again and again, which helps explain why these patients never seem to improve. Complicating this picture is the vulnerability of a fairly large portion of this patient population to chronic somatization.

Chronic somatization, as with somatization generally, represents a problem in ego functioning. Ego is a term that describes conscious executive functioning, such as planning, problem solving, and maintaining interpersonal relationships. As is discussed in chapter 6, somatizing patients have difficulty identifying and expressing emotions. Their considerable interpersonal ambivalence compromises the doctor-patient relationship and promotes high levels of dependency coupled with treatment-interfering behaviors. Despite their insistence that they want to be well, patients with chronic somatization actually rely on their condition for ego support; that is, somatization functions in the chronic population to provide ego stabilization. In the absence of ego integrative factors, patients with chronic somatization will manifest varying illness conditions despite effective symptomatic treatment.

With the situational patient, the picture is somewhat different. This population generally demonstrates a greater sense of ego organization. Situational subtypes can be employed in sometimes rather high level positions. They value independence, responsibility, and conformity to social norms. We encounter situational somatization when the patient is faced by an illness, surgical procedure, and the like, that carries the weight of an existential crisis. Although these patients rarely, if ever, verbalize their ambivalence in existential terms, somatization arises to protect the patient from disowned, unwanted, and unconscious personal traits. Shame figures largely in situational somatization particularly because illness and recovery entail dependence and a perceived loss of social status.

In both chronic and situational subtypes, progressive disorganization is a powerful factor. Progressive disorganization is a pre-psychotic process that results in a loss of the ability to function normally. Somatization literally "keeps the lid on" the chronic patient's tendency to decompensate under interpersonal pressures. While the situational subtype is not so vulnerable to pre-psychotic decompensation, the loss of functioning is tantamount to loss of one's self. Patients will go to great lengths to avoid the experience of disintegration, including withdrawing from treatment. It is an error to presume all patients possess normal ego functioning. True, the average patient wants to improve and return to daily life as quickly as possible. With somatization, however, we're dealing with a population that has serious ego impairment. Progressive disorganization can easily surface when we attempt to separate the patient from his or her source of ego support.

Mind-body integration is a subject of renewed interest in contemporary medical thinking and for good reason. Much of our training in the scientific method is rooted in an artificial distinction between mind and body that can be traced back more than one hundred years. Nevertheless, studies in the well-known placebo effect as well as the effects of psychotherapy on neuronal remodeling show how the mind, as both a conscious and unconscious entity, has the capacity to influence the body. Osteopathic medicine has long argued that alterations in visceral processing can result in somatic dysfunction and, conversely, somatic dysfunction can lead to visceral complications. In the case of the mind-body interface, rather than visceral-somatic or somato-visceral, we are describing cortico-somatic and cortico-visceral interactions. If it is possible for psychotherapy to produce changes in neural architecture, it is reasonable to conceptualize the development of physical pathology based on cortical processing. What the mind cannot express, the body will.

One of the most perplexing aspects of somatization is prediction. We know there is a rather high incidence of personality disorders in association with somatization, but that doesn't mean we must always find them together. Nor should we mistake malingering for somatization. Malingering is the conscious effort to feign illness for secondary gain. Somatization is an unconscious process that produces real physical symptomology, not uncommonly in the absence of biological markers. While empirical evidence for somatization can be obtained by administering a Paindex® test, as the senior author discovered, in the examination room the clinician depends on other factors to aid in diagnosis. Knowledge of the role of personality can serve as a very helpful and pragmatic tool in patient evaluation.

In the current volume we introduce the application of multilevel personality development to the somatization studies. Simply put, this means personality can be conceptualized by social, conscious, and unconscious dimensions. The social dimension is represented by the patient as seen by a fairly objective observer, namely, the clinician. The conscious dimension is the patient's self-report. It's a matter of how the patient is seen versus how they see themselves. Now, there may actually be quite a bit of difference between the observed personality and the self-report. Indeed, observed patient traits may lie completely outside their conscious awareness and when confronted with these differences, the patient may deny they exist. These represent unconscious elements which are manifest in behavior; they are known to observers and unknown to the individual. For example, a pleasant and affable patient seems a little annoyed and her remarks are harsh and accusatory. When the clinician suggests the patient might be angry, she denies ever feeling angry and insists she is just "preoccupied."

Among somatizing patients, we note four general personality types: managerial-autocratic, hypernormal, overly conventional, and dependent. Each of these types possesses specific and consistent traits that may point to a predisposition for either chronic or situational somatization. This is not to say that only these types are found among somatizers or that a hypernormal, for example, will always present with somatization. It does mean the collection of traits associated with each type tends to be found within the somatizing population. To this extent, they can be regarded as predictive; that is, when observed in a patient and coupled with a history of unexplained symptom complaints, complicated treatment response, and the like, one should seriously consider somatization in the differential diagnosis.

Because somatization represents a psychological problem, treatment ought to be, by definition, psychological. This is an important point and it should not be taken to mean a patient's physical condition isn't our concern; it should just not be the only concern. Under the pressure of patient demands for medical treatment, it is very easy to side step the real issue. This is rather like walking a tight rope: It's a skill that takes practice and when starting out, we're prone to falling. Eventually we learn to keep our eyes fixed on the goal and let balance take over. It's much like that when treating somatizing patients. We have to be sensitive to the fact that we are dealing with the mind-body interface and treatment needs to incorporate psychological as well as medical components. However, because somatizing patients present as chronic and situational, treatment needs to be tailored to type to be optimally effective. Behavioral therapies such as Cognitive-Behavioral Therapy, Cognitive-Behavioral Modification Therapy, and Dialectical Behavior Therapy have the potential to work well with the chronic subtype because these focus on empowering patients and teaching strategies for coping with and managing symptoms. One of the greatest barriers to psychological treatments of somatization is the patient's lack of psychological mindedness. Much like the physician who is ambivalent about mind-body interactions, somatizing patients argue their condition is solely physical and their mind has nothing to do with it. Psychological treatments are more effective when the patient is enlisted as an active partner and when treatments demonstrate the clinician's conviction that the patient's condition is not imaginary.

Situational somatization, because it relates to experiences that carry the weight of an existential crisis, should be treated with short-term existential psychotherapy. While therapy for the chronic subtype is directed toward improving ego functioning within the limits of patient tolerance, existential psychotherapy is an indirect approach to somatization. Rather than confronting the patient's ego defenses and attending to the illness condition, the existential therapist circumvents the patient's symptoms and addresses the existential crisis that lies at the heart of her distress. By resolving the crisis that stimulates the need for somatization, we lessen, and hopefully eliminate, the patient's reliance upon it. We suggest that short-term, goal-oriented existential therapy is preferable because even the situational population has a limited capacity to remain in treatment. The likelihood of patients completing treatment is increased when the end is always kept in sight.

Psychopharmacology poses interesting clinical problems. The results of clinical trials are mixed and no particular class of medications or any individual medication has been shown to have a reliably robust effect upon somatization. If there is evidence of comorbid depression or anxiety, we can certainly make that a focus of treatment. With somatization, however, pharmacological interventions are not always straightforward and clinical judgment has to take center stage when deciding whether or not to prescribe. The obvious question we must ask is: How do you get a patient to take psychiatric medications for a condition they argue is purely physical? The answer to this lies in the doctor-patient relationship. As with any sort of pharmacotherapy, compliance is dependent on many factors including the patient's expectation of relief, frequency of dosage, the doctor's confidence in the efficacy of the medication and, above all, the patient's belief that the doctor has his or her best interests in mind. A treatment alliance with somatizing patients is difficult to achieve and even more difficult to maintain. Nevertheless, we argue that a supportive relationship with the patient has the greatest likelihood of ensuring compliance, even with this patient population.

Working with both chronic and situational subtypes is demanding and can seem daunting, particularly when the clinician relies on conventional thinking about the mind-body interface. Patients demand time that is in short supply in our current managed health care environment. Clinicians are frustrated by uncertain diagnoses, poor outcomes, and recalcitrant patients. There is tremendous potential for the clinician to find a renewed sense of hope and empathy for this population. Achieving this requires changing one's outlook on mind-body interactions, learning how to identify somatization and developing an active understanding of the role it plays in patients' lives. We are far more likely to adjust our expectations than our patients but when we undertake the task, there is a good chance we will make a difference in their quality of life. And, after all, isn't that why we entered medicine in the first place?

OUTLINE OF CHAPTERS

Chapter 1 is divided into two sections. Part 1 briefly develops the history of current diagnostic thinking about somatization as it is represented by the DSM. Part 2 is devoted to a detailed discussion of the DSM somatoform disorders as well as a number of dimensional classification alternatives.

In chapter 2 we discuss difficulties involved in somatization studies, particularly the discontent experienced by clinicians, patients, and managed care. We suggest that a more enlightened approach can be helpful, one involving personality traits as well as biological, social, and cultural factors.

Chapter 3 develops the concept of clinician ambivalence with respect to somatization. To a great extent, this involves a misunderstanding of the mind-body interface which is a direct outgrowth of the nature of our scientific training. Drawing upon the placebo effect and neuroscientific studies of psychotherapy, we argue that the mind-body interface is a critical element in the evaluation and treatment of the somatizing patient.

Chapter 4 highlights the role of ambivalence and progressive disorganization. As previously stated, ambivalence in somatization is both interpersonal and intrapersonal, and represents a key element in the patient's ego structure. Progressive disorganization constitutes a powerful threat to ego integrity. For the chronic subtype, somatization serves as a focus about which ego functions are organized. In the case of the situational subtype, somatization represents the ultimate defense against ego disintegration.

Chapter 5 further develops the themes of perception and multilevel perceptual diagnosis in somatization. Just as the resolution of ambivalence requires us to reconcile opposing emotions, appearance and interpretation must be united in order to accurately perceive existential reality. The inability to do so is a neurotic process and can be observed in somatization. When we respond to another person with a sense of inexplicable revulsion, interpretation is divorced from appearance and our feelings reflect unconscious projection rather than a reality-based, existential perception of the person. Either one represses the event or the meaning assigned to it; in either case, the repressed material tends to become dominant in the psychological makeup of the person. In somatization, the dominant unconscious element becomes an unconscious pattern of somatic displacement.

The second half of chapter 5 focuses on the use of a system of multilevel perceptual diagnosis in clinical decision making. The concept of multilevel diagnosis is based upon Leary's interpersonal theory of personality, which describes how personality functions between discrete, yet interdependent, levels. Utilizing the Paindex® test and the SDA Screen®, the authors discuss how intrapersonal conflict may be objectively determined and evaluated within the somatization process.

Confronting and coping with impasse resistance in the somatizing patient is a challenging and frequently daunting task. Chapter 6 applies the concept of multilevel diagnosis by outlining specific personality types which most often present in the clinical setting with somatization-related symptom complaints.

Chapters 7 through 9 address critical issues of treatment with respect to somatizing patients. Chapter 7 discusses the role of Cognitive-Behavior as well as Cognitive-Behavior Modification Therapy in the treatment of chronic somatization. Chapter 8 examines Dialectical Behavior Therapy and its applicability to the chronic population. In chapter 9, the theory and practice of existential psychotherapy is introduced as a unique treatment option for patients diagnosed with situational somatization.

Chapter 10 discusses psychopharmacological interventions for the somatizing patient and focuses on clinical applications derived from practice management and direct patient contact. Data supportive for antidepressant treatment is mixed and benzodiazepines have limited utility. This chapter focuses on clinical applications derived from practice management and direct patient contact.

Chapter 11 summarizes the material presented and reiterates the value of existential theory in the evaluation and treatment of the somatizing patient.

Chapter One

Somatization and the Power of Conventional Wisdom

It has been long recognized that emotional stress exerts a powerful influence on physical health while physical illness strongly influences psychological and emotional health. Some patients, in fact, seem more inclined to experience and communicate emotional distress in physical, rather than emotional, terms.[1] Characteristically, individuals who experience and communicate emotional and psychological distress as symptoms of a medical illness tend to report a degree of pain, discomfort, and incapacitation that is out of proportion to physical and laboratory findings. We describe these persons as having a somatization syndrome. Somatization is reported as one of the most common illnesses encountered by primary care physicians and is generally associated with a disproportionately high number of physician visits, subsequent laboratory investigations, drug prescriptions, and surgical interventions.[2] It is estimated that in the United States alone, 10 percent of medical services are delivered to patients with no demonstrable evidence of organic disease, and at a cost estimated at $20 billion annually.[3] During 1989, 25 percent of cumulative trauma disorders reported in the United States accounted for 80 percent of the estimated $563 million paid in compensation. In the same year, cases of "soft tissue" back and neck pain were reported to account for 45 percent of all workers compensation payments and 39 percent of all hospitalizations.[4] Somatizing syndromes exert a powerful impact on the workplace.

Despite the prevalence of somatizing syndromes, there tends to be an absence of complete agreement among medical and psychological practitioners as to their diagnosis and treatment. Although the Diagnostic and Statistical Manual of Mental Disorders (DSM) is generally regarded as the gold standard for psychiatric diagnosis, it can be argued that its approach to somatizing syndromes is neither extensive nor absolute. In this chapter, we shall examine the current diagnostic evaluations of somatization with particular attention to the DSM categories and alternative/supplementary approaches suggested in the professional literature. We encourage the reader who is familiar with psychiatric terminology and diagnostic procedures to read on; in our experience, it isn't the case that one may have had too much exposure to these concepts, but rather, far too little.

THE DSM AND DIAGNOSTIC CLASSIFICATION

Seventy-five years ago, psychiatric researchers realized that a new and more comprehensive conceptual framework was needed to make sense of the vast array of persons who complained of physical symptoms in the absence of apparent physical disease. Wilhelm Stekel, the physician who essentially invented the term "somatization" in 1924, described it as "a bodily disorder that arises as an expression of deep-seated neurosis"; that is, mental anguish, not consciously acknowledged, may manifest itself as physical complaints.[5] Stekel's conceptualization gave rise to the whole spectrum of psychosomatic disorders, the treatment of which was largely psychoanalytic in approach. Over the years, most of Stekel's diagnostic terms have fallen by the wayside, although one remains in our clinical vernacular: hypochondriasis. Clearly an old clinical problem, somatization is formally included in the DSM under the rubric of Somatization Disorder within the overall category of somatoform disorders. Other somatoform diagnoses include Undifferentiated Somatoform Disorder, Conversion Disorder, Body Dysmorphic Disorder, Pain Disorder, Hypochondriasis, and Somatoform Disorder Not Otherwise Specified.[6] While these share some common features, we know that somatic symptoms are so ubiquitous that it is almost impossible to separate psychiatric illness from what may be a temporary retreat from conflict and stress.[7] By improving the diagnostic terms applicable to the somatizing patient, we gain new understanding into the essential fact that disorders related to somatization do not necessarily involve conscious intent.[8]

Looking back over the past century and a half, it is safe to say that Emil Kraepelin is frequently regarded as the father of modern psychiatric diagnosis. Writing during the latter part of the nineteenth century, Kraepelin began his work as reaction against the biological psychiatry of the time.[9]

> The biological psychiatrists had spawned a sprawl of clinical disease labels, each based on the particular circumstances associated with an illness ("masturbatory insanity," "wedding night psychosis") or on the particular combination of symptoms ("chronic delusional disorder"), with almost no correlation to brain

> pathology. Multi-infarct dementia, neurosyphilis, thyroid deficiency, and the like were the only exceptions.[10]

Over the course of successive editions of his psychiatric textbook, Kraepelin attempted to classify diseases by observing symptoms. In the 1896 edition, he stated that he was weary of this approach and rather than try to determine the causes of illness, he began to focus his attention on the prediction of outcomes.[11] For Kraepelin, "the value of a diagnosis for the practical activity of the psychiatrist consists of letting him give a reliable look at the future."[12] As a consequence of his change of direction, the interpretation of symptoms would ultimately become less important than their observation and description. The DSM is the modern heir to the revolution in diagnostic procedures initiated by Kraepelin.

The DSM IV-TR (2003) is regarded by many as the most ambitious project in the American Psychiatric Association's history of defining diagnostic nomenclature. A revision of the DSM-IV (1994), the DSM-IV-TR is the most recent volume in a history that includes the DSM-III-R (1987), the DSM III (1980), DSM-II (1968), and, finally, the DSM-I (1952). The first editions of the DSM were created in response to the need for uniform diagnostic standards for psychological conditions. Criticisms related to low validity and reliability in these earlier versions led to the development of the DSM-III, which represented the beginning of the American Psychiatric Association's efforts to increase diagnostic validity and reliability by means of a more descriptive approach that linked diagnoses to research findings.[13] Additional changes, including the multiaxial system whereby patients are diagnosed along five axis, marked the DSM-III and DSM-III-R. The multiaxial system represents the attempt to situate primary Axis I diagnoses such as schizophrenia within a biopsychosocial context. Personality disorders and mental retardation are indicated on Axis II, biological factors on Axis III, psychosocial stressors on Axis IV, and an overall global assessment of functioning rated numerically on a scale of 1 to 100 on Axis V. Despite these changes, neither volume was accepted with complete satisfaction. There was widespread criticism, for example, that the DSM-III and DSM-III-R masked an implicit "medical model of psychopathology, which places the diagnosis and treatment of psychopathology firmly in the field of the psychiatric profession to the exclusion of psychologists, social workers, and other mental health professionals."[14] Some argued that these volumes relied too heavily on a categorical approach whereby a patient either does or does not have a particular disorder; these criticisms have been leveled by many against newer editions of the DSM as well.[15]

An essentially practical manual, the DSM is designed to produce a taxonomy of mental disorders, classifying them in much the same way as are biological organisms by the familiar categories of kingdom, phylum, class, order, family, genus, and species that every biology 101 student is required to memorize. The beauty of this approach lies in the fact that it is relatively easy to learn and apply in clinical situations. Smaller versions of the DSM, comprised solely of diagnostic criteria, find their way into the white coats of medical students during their psychiatric rotations. Patients who ask for a formal psychological explanation for their condition are often given handouts which reflect DSM terminology. The DSM provides clinicians with a kind of diagnostic shorthand that facilitates efficient communication. Researchers base inclusion/exclusion criteria on its diagnostic formulations. Managed care organizations require DSM or ICD-10 (International Classification of Disorders, Revision 10) diagnostic codes when billing for services rendered. In short, the DSM tends to dominate the way in which we conceptualize psychopathology in the twenty-first century.

One of the most notable features of successive versions of the DSM is length. Since its inception, the DSM has grown to comprise more than 800 pages. To a certain extent, this makes sense. As our knowledge of psychopathology becomes more extensive, it's reasonable the catalog would grow proportionately. Not everyone agrees with this proposition, however. Houts, for example, argues that the proliferation of DSM diagnoses indicates we are becoming less adept at conceptualizing psychopathology rather than more.[16] Scientific progress takes place when more general explanations are developed to account for observed phenomena.

> Specifically with regard to taxonomy, progress occurred when classification systems were reduced by the innovation of a theory to account for the variety of observations. For example, primitive biological knowledge was organized in terms of description and categorization based on surface features of organisms. Before Charles Darwin, complex taxonomies emerged and the number of categories needed to account for living things proliferated. With the rise of evolutionary theory in the twentieth century, classification in terms of surface features was replaced by classification based on phylogenetic and, later, genetic concepts. The role of taxonomy changed from one of storing and retrieving information to one of providing evidence for a theory of origins. Taxonomies no longer did the job of explaining, but instead became the thing to be explained. According to this model, scientific progress occurs when there is a reduction by theory of the number of taxonomic categories; the mere proliferation of categories is sure sign that progress has not, in fact, occurred.[17]

Accordingly, despite claims that expansions of DSM diagnostic categories reflect scientific progress, these claims are, in fact, inconsistent with the traditional model of scientific progress.[18] When the appeal is made to the analogy from physical medicine—that is, increased knowledge of disease processes naturally leads to increased specificity in diagnostic labels— Houts replies that the modern disease nomenclature reflected in the ICD series has actually produced a reduction in disease labels.[19] Developments in clinical microbiology, for example, have reduced the domain of illnesses which are solely classified by symptom topography.[20] Appealing to Scadding's Ladder of Medical Disorder Diagnostic Knowledge, Houts points out that as scientific knowledge increases, the progression moves away from syndromal classification towards etiology.[21] Following this line of thinking, progress in psychiatric diagnosis does not occur when we see a proliferation of diagnostic categories as is observed in the DSM, but rather when syndromally defined disorders are reduced by an explanation of their etiology.[22]

To the credit of the DSM committee, not every suggested diagnosis finds its way into print—some are given provisionary status. Examples of the latter include Intermittent Explosive Disorder and Paranoid Personality Disorder. Several factors underlie the development of multiple diagnostic labels. First, a diagnosis provides a solution to social problems.[23] Individuals frequently come to the attention of mental health clinicians because their behavior has resulted in some measure of interpersonal distress or disturbance. Application of a diagnosis provides an explanation that carries the weight of authority and offers hope for change. A diagnosis may offer an individual the possibility of obtaining social services or alleviate the social stigma attached to certain kinds of behaviors. In any case, the "more diagnoses we have at our disposal, the more options we have to bring relief to those who benefit from including disturbing behavior under the authority and sanction of mental health practitioners."[24] Second, the availability of diagnostic categories provides the clinician with relief from professional discomfort.[25] When faced with a patient in distress, clinicians tend to feel more competent when able to place the patient's condition within specific categories of dysfunction. This, in turn, reinforces the patient's faith in the practitioner and, hopefully, increases the likelihood of treatment compliance.

Some diagnoses serve an additional function of actually suggesting lines of treatment. For example, the psychotic symptoms of schizophrenia, assuming they have been ruled out as indicative of organic disease or other factors, direct the practitioner to the prescription of neuroleptic medication. From a very practical standpoint, a diagnosis provides the practitioner with the clinical justification for seeking payment from managed care providers.

Diagnostic categories also render research easier to conduct and support.[26] Researchers can more readily identify potential populations for study when an established diagnostic category provides inclusion/exclusion criteria. The expansion of diagnoses "extends the practice of diagnosis to include more and more human behaviors, thereby extending the scope of research that is acceptable, publishable, and fundable."[27]

Finally, the proliferation of diagnoses can be understood as a marketing tool.[28] On the one hand, pharmaceutical companies benefit from having new opportunities to apply their products, particularly when marketing targets the consumer. We have all seen television advertisements which conclude, "Ask your doctor if xyz medication is right for you." Others include the all-too-familiar terms, "chemical imbalance," which tends to convey the message that psychopathology is primarily a biological phenomena which submits primarily to pharmaceutical interventions. Thus, not only is a particular diagnosis marketed to the public, but it also represents a particular view about the nature of mental disorders.[29] Ultimately, as diagnostic labels increase in number, the need for newer editions of the DSM and DSM-related materials is generated and the whole process of marketing psychopathology comes full circle. It would be a serious error, of course, to regard these elements as the sole motivating factors for the development of new diagnostic categories, but a critical discussion requires their mention.

One of the characteristics of categorical approaches to species organization is the presence of prototypical members and fuzzy boundaries.[30] This is precisely the case with the DSM. For example, the prototypic patient with schizophrenia has evidence of hallucinations and psychotic thought processes in the absence of symptoms of a Mood Disorder. The prototypic patient with a Mood Disorder has evidence of depression or mania in the absence of symptoms of psychosis. Yet, there are patients who present with symptoms of both Schizophrenia and a Mood Disorder. The DSM allows for this kind of diagnostic variance by providing the diagnostic category of Schizoaffective Disorder. The blurring of categorical boundaries becomes more acute in the case of personality disorders where it is more difficult to distinguish between normal and pathological behaviors. Thus, we are often faced with diagnostic uncertainty. Patients may present with symptoms of a disorder yet fail to meet full criteria for a diagnosis. They may also meet diagnostic criteria for more than one disorder in the same category or possess symptoms for more than one psychiatric disorder at the same time. Comorbidity thus becomes an important factor to consider. The DSM provides guidelines rather than strict rules for resolving diagnostic uncertainty and we do well to remind ourselves that this process is more art than science.

Nevertheless, some authors argue that diagnostic uncertainty derives, to a certain extent, from the mistake of applying a categorical approach to every problem of psychopathology. Joiner and Schmidt argue "for an approach that allows us to distinguish empirically between syndromes best described as categories and those better described as dimensions."[31] As we stated above, a categorical approach indicates that a patient either has or does not have a particular disorder. But patients are people and often fail to cooperate with our diagnostic efforts by falling neatly into one category or another. Rather than attempting to solve the problem of fuzzy boundaries by developing a midrange category such as Schizoaffective Disorder to account for overlapping symptoms, Joiner and Schmidt wonder if psychopathological syndromes can be more accurately regarded as "graded, dimensional continua, along which everybody can be placed, ranging from those with absent or minimal symptoms, on up to those with very severe symptoms."[32] The difficulty with both categorical and dimensional approaches is the absence of definitive empirical evidence compelling us to go either way. This dilemma can be solved, the authors state, by utilizing an approach called taxometrics that was developed by Paul E. Meehl.[33] Taxometrics is an analytical system that determines whether a thing is, or is not, a taxon. The term "taxon" refers to something that is one thing and not another. A Chevrolet Corvette, an obstetrician, a bassoon player are examples of taxa. Nontaxa are more variable and by default belong to dimensional continua, such as height, weight, blood pressure, and the like.

Rather than describe taxometrics in detail, we will give an example of how it works. Beginning with a taxon and some indicators associated with it, such as depression with sadness, anhedonia, and suicidality, we assign scores to a group of individuals along each indicator according to the severity of symptom complaint, let's say, from 1 to 7. The next step involves examining the correlations between two indicators against a third.

> If depression is a taxon, two indicators (e.g., sadness and anhedonia) will correlate negligibly at the low end of the third indicator (e.g., among those who score 1 on suicidality), where the majority of taxon nonmembers would be. The two indicators will correlate more and more highly as the midrange of the third indicator is approached (where the mixture of taxon members and nonmembers would peak), and will correlate negligibly at the high end of the third indicator (where the majority of taxon members would be). If depression is not a taxon, but rather is a dimensional continuum, the intercorrelation of any two indicators will not systematically vary as a function of a third indicator.[34]

The data is then graphed to facilitate the observation of peaks; a series of peaked graphs indicate taxonicity and flat graphs, dimensionality. There is quite a bit more to taxometrics, including consistency checks and the evaluation of indicators to determine which ones are good markers of a taxon, but for our purposes, it is sufficient to see how the process is undertaken. Although clinicians are hardly expected to use taxometrics, for the researcher, it can be a valuable tool for diagnostic clarification, and if we are going to grant any credence to the idea of dimensional approaches to psychopathology, it's going to be important to have an analytic tool that permits us to empirically determine what should and should not be considered a category.

Dimensional approaches have been proposed in other contexts. Akiskal, for example, argues that Bipolar Disorder can be more accurately understood in terms of a "bipolarity spectrum," than simply the diagnostic categories of the DSM. Instead of the familiar Bipolar I and Bipolar II disorders which, respectively, present alternating episodes of mania/hypomania and depression, Akiskal draws upon the clinical literature to elucidate four developing subtypes of Bipolar Disorder. These "softer" variants of bipolarity present a much more complicated clinical picture of the condition than was previously imagined. The difficulty with the descriptions given bipolarity in the DSM relate to its atheoretical approach:

> The atheoretical position of the DSM-IV diagnostic system may serve as a blueprint for a research document, but regrettably it does not do justice to the clinical complexity of bipolarity as seen by the practitioner; nor does the DSM-IV provide any guidance for how to make sense of the conditions that accompany bipolar illness. Reformulating Bipolar Disorder as a spectrum has clinically meaningful implications for comorbidity, the nature of a putative shared underlying pathophysiology, clinical management, and public health.[35]

According to Akiskal, the prototypic descriptions of Bipolar Disorder in the DSM should serve more as guidelines directing the clinician toward the most likely diagnosis of "an elusive and complex array of affective manifestations subthreshold to the classical bipolar type."[36]

In his discussion of schizophrenia, Tsuang points out that the DSM describes this disorder as a discrete diagnostic category rather than a quantitative dimension.[37] The problem with this approach is "a reliance on discrete categories raises potential problems for cases that share symptoms of multiple disorders because they may lead to artificial boundary categories and elevated rates of comorbidity."[38] Although dimensional models are imperfect, Tsuang believes a dimensional approach has some distinct advantages for thinking about schizophrenia. For one thing, dimensional models allow for persons who possess varying degrees of risk factors for the disorder: "People with very high doses (of risk factors) are at high risk for schizophrenia; those with moderate doses may have related conditions such as Schizotypal Personality Disorder, negative symptoms, neurophysiological impairment, or other neurobiological manifestations of the predisposition to schizophrenia."[39] In a sense, rather than viewing schizophrenia as the prototypical diagnostic category, Tsuang calls attention to the term "schizotaxia" which has been proposed to describe the unexpressed genetic predisposition to schizophrenia. Individuals with schizotaxia may go on to develop schizotypy or schizophrenia, depending on the liability or protection afforded by environmental cicumstances.[40] There is a great deal of interest in the psychiatric literature about treating prodromal symptoms of schizophrenia in the hope of improving overall outcomes.[41] From a dimensional point of view, we are actually dealing with schizotaxia in the case of persons who present with prodromal symptomology.

> It will become useful to change our conceptualization of schizophrenia somewhat from the historical view of a discrete, categorical entity whose diagnosis depended on the clinical symptoms of psychosis. Instead, a more fruitful approach may be to incorporate a dimensional, neurodevelopmental perspective on schizophrenia that includes neurobiological and neurophysiological measures occurring prior to the development of psychosis (schizotaxia).[42]

Dimensional approaches permit the kind of flexibility that is necessary for evaluating subtle syndromal distinctions and the impact on clinical work can be significant.

Variations on the dimensional approach also appear in the literature on somatization. The popularity and clinical utility of the DSM, however, renders it essential to understand somatization within this context as well. As we have stated previously, contemporary psychiatric diagnosis tends to follow the DSM and conventional wisdom can be a very powerful thing. For this reason, the next section is devoted to the DSM criteria for somatizing syndromes as well as a discussion of alternatives to this approach and their advantages and disadvantages.

SOMATOFORM DISORDERS AND FUNCTIONAL SOMATIC SYNDROMES

The overall subject heading of Somatoform Disorders brings together a group of disorders that are suggestive of a general medical condition, yet are not fully explained by one.[43] Briefly, the somatoform disorders can be described thusly:

Somatization Disorder (historically referred to as hysteria or Briquet's syndrome) is a polysymptomatic disorder that begins before age 30, extends over a period of years, and is characterized by a combination of pain, gastrointestinal, sexual, and pseudoneurological symptoms.

Undifferentiated Somatoform Disorder is characterized by unexplained physical complaints, lasting at least six months, that are below the threshold for a diagnosis of Somatization Disorder.

Conversion Disorder involves unexplained symptoms or deficits affecting voluntary motor or sensory function that suggests a neurological or other general medical condition. Psychological factors are judged to be associated with the symptoms or deficits.

Pain Disorder is characterized by pain as the predominant focus of clinical attention. In addition, psychological factors are judged to have an important role in its onset, severity, exacerbation, or maintenance.

Hypochondriasis is the preoccupation with the fear of having, or the idea that one has, a serious disease based on the person's misinterpretation of bodily symptoms or bodily functions.

Body Dysmorphic Disorder is the preoccupation with an imagined or exaggerated defect in physical appearance.

Somatoform Disorder Not Otherwise Specified is included for coding disorders with somatoform symptoms that do not meet the criteria for any of the specific somatoform disorders.[44]

Under the general Somatoform rubric are three diagnostic syndromes specific to somatization: Somatization Disorder, Undifferentiated Somatoform Disorder, and Somatoform Disorder NOS (Not Otherwise Specified). Typically, somatizing conditions are diagnosed with one of these three categories. The question of whether, or to what extent, Conversion Disorder, Body Dysmorphic Disorder, and Hypochondriasis qualify as somatization disorders will be left until later in this section when dimensional approaches are discussed. Arguably, Pain Disorder Associated with Psychological Factors may also be regarded as a somatizing syndrome insofar as psychological factors are considered important in the onset, severity, exacerbation, or maintenance of the reported pain.[45] Nevertheless, because painful symptoms are often associated with Somatization Disorder, Undifferentiated Somatoform Disorder, and Somatoform Disorder NOS, we will focus on the diagnostic criteria for each of these in turn, beginning with Somatization Disorder.

300.81: Somatization Disorder[46]

A. A history of many physical complaints beginning before age 30 that occur over a period of several years and result in treatment being sought or significant impairment in social, occupational, or other important areas of functioning.

B. Each of the following criteria must have been met, with individual symptoms occurring at any time during the course of the disturbance:

(1) four pain symptoms: a history of pain related to at least four different sites or functions (e.g., head, abdomen, back, joints, extremities, chest, rectum, during menstruation, during sexual intercourse, or during urination)

(2) two gastrointestinal symptoms: a history of two gastrointestinal symptoms other than pain (e.g., nausea, bloating, vomiting other than during pregnancy, diarrhea, or intolerance of several different foods)

(3) one sexual symptom: a history of at least one sexual or reproductive symptom other than pain (e.g., sexual indifference, erectile or ejaculatory dysfunction, irregular menses, excessive menstrual bleeding, vomiting throughout pregnancy)
(4) one pseudoneurological symptom: a history of at least one symptom or deficit suggesting a neurological condition not limited to pain (conversion symptoms such as impaired coordination or balance, paralysis or localized weakness, difficulty swallowing or lump in the throat, aphonia, urinary retention, hallucinations, loss of touch or pain sensation, double vision, blindness, deafness, seizures, dissociative symptoms such as amnesia, or loss of consciousness other than fainting)

C. Either (1) or (2):

(1) after appropriate investigation, each of the symptoms in Criterion B cannot be fully explained by a known general medical condition or the direct effects of a substance (e.g., a drug of abuse, a medication)
(2) when there is a related general medical condition, the physical complaints of resulting social or occupational impairment are in excess of what would be expected from the history, physical examination, or laboratory findings

D. The symptoms are not intentionally produced or feigned (as in Factitious Disorder or Malingering).

Somatization Disorder is "a pattern of recurring, multiple, clinically significant somatic complaints," and represents a chronic condition marked by a minimum of eight symptoms from four symptom categories, the presence of which cannot be attributed to a general medical condition or the direct effects of a substance.[47] According to the DSM writers, the illness complaints of persons with Somatization Disorder are frequently exaggerated and supporting factual information is often lacking.[48] These patients tend to be poor historians and, as a consequence of having sought treatment from more than one physician, may have histories of "complicated and sometimes hazardous combinations of treatments."[49] Their clinical picture may be complicated by comorbid mood and/or anxiety symptoms as well as features of personality disorders. The course of Somatization Disorder may be marked by periods of remission, but rarely does an individual experience a single year without some kind of somatic complaint prompting medical attention.[50]

Due to the number and variety of symptoms required to meet criteria for Somatization Disorder, most somatizing patients are diagnosed with Undifferentiated Somatoform Disorder.[51]

300.82 Undifferentiated Somatoform Disorder[52]

A. One or more physical complaints (e.g., fatigue, loss of appetite, gastrointestinal or urinary complaints).

B. Either (1) or (2):

(1) after appropriate investigation, the symptoms cannot be fully explained by a known general medical condition or the direct effects of a substance (e.g., a drug of abuse, a medication)
(2) when there is a related general medical condition, the physical complaints or resulting social or occupational impairment is in excess of what would be expected from the history, physical examination, or laboratory findings

C. The symptoms cause clinically significant distress or impairment in social, occupational, or other important areas of functioning.

D. The duration of the disturbance is at least six months.

E. The disturbance is not better accounted for by another mental disorder (e.g., another Somatoform Disorder, Sexual Dysfunction, Mood Disorder, Anxiety Disorder, Sleep Disorder, or Psychotic Disorder).

F. The symptom is not intentionally produced or feigned (as in Factitious Disorder or Malingering).

Aside from the number and kinds of symptoms required to meet criteria for a diagnosis, Undifferentiated Somatoform Disorder is also distinguished from Somatization Disorder by the length of time symptomology must be present. Somatic symptoms of duration less than six months must be diagnosed as the Undifferentiated type.

300.82 Somatoform Disorder Not Otherwise Specified[53]

This category includes disorders with somatoform symptoms that do not meet the criteria for any specific Somatoform Disorder. Examples include:

1. Pseudocyesis: a false belief of being pregnant that is associated with objective signs of pregnancy, which may include abdominal enlargement (although the umbilicus does not become everted), reduced menstrual flow, amenorrhea, subjective sensation of fetal movement, nausea, breast engorgement and secretions, and labor pains at the expected date of delivery. Endocrine changes may be present, but the syndrome cannot be explained by a general medical condition that causes endocrine changes (e.g., a hormone-secreting tumor).
2. A disorder involving nonpsychotic hypochondriacal symptoms of less than six months' duration.

3. A disorder involving unexplained physical complaints (e.g., fatigue or body weakness) of less than six months' duration that are not due to another mental disorder.

The NOS, or "not otherwise specified," category is one that appears in each diagnostic group within the DSM and serves as a catch-all diagnosis when patients fail to meet criteria for a more specific disorder. Thus, this category represents one way of solving the problem of diagnostic uncertainty and "essentially plugs gaps in the diagnostic system and ensures there will be a diagnosis, albeit at the least common denominator, for any patient who exhibits the predominant symptoms of a diagnostic group . . . even if their clinical presentation is atypical."[54] Accordingly, the Somatoform Disorder NOS category can be a very useful one, especially for symptoms that appear to be of fairly recent onset (less than six months).

The guidelines operative in these three categories exemplify the model followed throughout the DSM. Exclusion criteria serve to isolate a psychiatric disorder from a general medical one or the influence of pharmacology and/or drugs of abuse. The individual categories themselves serve to distinguish the polysymptomatic and chronic Somatization Disorder from conditions of more recent onset with fewer or, perhaps, more targeted physical complaints.

Due to its relatively straightforward presentation, familiar approach to classification, and apparent usefulness, one might imagine the DSM's popularity virtually dismisses any further discussion of diagnostic nosology. We have a classification system that has gained widespread acceptance, and that, as they say, is that. Nevertheless, as we pointed out earlier, there are distinct problems with the DSM and its approach to somatization.

To begin with, some authors question whether the DSM's categorical organization of somatoform disorders accurately represents the nature of these disorders. For example, Escobar et al. suggest that somatoform disorders might actually lie along a somatoform continuum rather than specifying discrete diagnostic species.[55] Utilizing a dimensional, rather than a descriptive model, Somatization Disorder would be placed at the "severe" end of the spectrum and Hypochondriasis, Undifferentiated Somatoform Disorder, Somatoform Disorder NOS, and the like, would represent less severe or evolving forms of pathology.[56] In part, Escobar et al. based this idea on observations that Somatization Disorder proper tends to have a lower incidence than sub-syndromal forms, further suggesting the possibility of an "abridged somatization disorder."[57] Allen et al. note that "abridged somatization is widespread in primary care and is associated with high rates of disability, medical utilization, and psychiatric comorbidity."[58] In addition, unlike Somatization Disorder, which has a low incidence among males in the United States, the Allen et al. study showed the debilitation that accompanies somatization affects both men and women when somatization is defined by the abridged criteria (four or more unexplained medical symptoms in men and six or more in women).[59]

Robbins and Kirmayer develop a more inclusive concept that integrates varieties of somatic concern under the broad umbrella of somatization, which is then divided into three subtypes. In the tradition of descriptive psychiatric epidemiology, somatization refers

> to the number of medically unexplained or functional somatic symptoms during one's lifetime. We have called this functional somatization. In the study of clinical illness behavior, somatization refers to the worry or belief that one has or is vulnerable to a serious illness despite reassurances from physicians and the absence of demonstrable disease. We have called this form hypochondriacal somatization. In the tradition of studies of mental disorders in primary care, somatization refers to the presentation of exclusively somatic symptoms to the general practitioner despite the presence of psychiatric illness. We have called this last form presenting somatization.[60]

Citing sociodemographic profiles as well as cognitive and perceptual factors associated with each subtype, these authors describe somatization in a way they believe has been relatively neglected in the scholarly literature. There is a tendency, they say, for writers to make unwarranted assumptions that characteristics of one form of somatization apply equally to others, hence the necessity of clarifying each concept in order to facilitate a better understanding of the processes involved in what they regard as distinct forms of somatization.[61]

It is worthy to note that Robbins and Kirmayer do not conceptualize somatization in terms of DSM categories; instead, they focus on the characteristics of each type utilizing a more dimensional approach and present somatization as an overarching phenomenon that is encountered in three forms in the clinical setting. The first type, functional somatization, seems to encompass those conditions which qualify for a diagnosis of either Somatization Disorder or Allen's Abridged Somatization Disorder. Hypochondriacal somatization reflects their belief that hypochondriasis is a distinct form of somatization and that illness complaints are often encountered in the absence of physical symptoms.[62] Presenting somatization describes the patient who seeks medical care primarily for somatic concerns but is also found to have a psychiatric condition, that is, a mood or anxiety disorder, that may account for their symptoms.[63]

One of the difficulties with Robbins and Kirmayer's approach is the absence of a clear definition of somatization. If we read them correctly, it seems they are working from the perspective that somatization reflects a pathological concern about physical symptomology. Whether that concern is the result of disease phobia, psychiatric illness, or unexplained symptoms, and thus falls under one of their subtypes, the overall process is called somatization. While we applaud their efforts to define somatization dimensionally, we are concerned, nevertheless, that they may have overgeneralized the concept. From our perspective, somatization is a technical term which specifically describes the disease process in terms of the mind-body interface. As such, it is important to distinguish between somatization and hypochondriasis, for example. To their credit, Robbins and Kirmayer note Kellner's objection that, while functional somatic symptoms and hypochondriasis often appear together in studies, they are in fact, different phenomena, a position echoed by Liebrand and Hiller.[64] In his 1992 study of forty-two hypochondriacal patients, Barsky noted that, while one-fifth of those patients studied also qualified for Somatization Disorder, hypochondriasis and somatization nonetheless seemed "phenomenologically distinct."[65] In our experience, there is a clear, conscious element in the ruminations of hypochondriacal patients that may suggest secondary and/or tertiary gain, while among somatizers, the disease phobia seems largely absent and physical complaints are powerfully driven by unconscious factors.

Regarding their subtype of psychiatric somatization, Robbins and Kirmayer cite Bridges and Goldberg who distinguish between facultative and true somatizers; the "former acknowledged psychological distress when skillfully interviewed, while the latter persisted in rejecting any psychological attribution for their symptoms."[66] Given the current interest in the psychiatric literature regarding physical symptoms associated with mood disorders, Robbins and Kirmayer make a valid point, namely, that some physical complaints are related to certain Axis I disorders.[67] Nevertheless, we are uncomfortable with the use of the word "somatization" in this context as well. Why not simply state that some patients experience physical distress in association with a mood disorder? Describing their condition as a type of somatization is confusing, to our way of thinking, and leads the clinician to introduce diagnostic considerations that might well be foreign to the patient's presentation.

A further difficulty with the DSM's approach to somatization lies in the fact that it perpetuates what we believe is the fallacious notion that mind and body are unrelated entities. In this regard Martin argues that the apparent disinterest in physiology on the part of the DSM committee results in physical symptom complaints being traceable only to psychological issues.[68] More important, he states,

> there is an implied abhorrence of the idea that psychosomatic causality may play a role in the patients seen under the somatoform rubric. Psychosomatic causality is the concept that mind-body interactions are responsible for disease production. Its opposite would be the contention that mind or body, alone, separate, apart, is operating in an individual manner to give its own group of disorders.[69]

As a result, there are mind-related illnesses and body-related illnesses and neither can interact with or affect the other: "Mind problems do not cause body problems . . . body problems do not cause mind problems."[70] The approach of the DSM is simply the observation of presenting symptoms and categorization according to similarity. Causal and descriptive ideas are thus viewed as incongruent.[71] The outcome of this situation is what Martin describes as a conundrum:

> If one remains purely descriptive and concedes to an official somatoform diagnosis, causal factors are presumed irrelevant. Unknown does not mean irrelevant. If causal factors are relegated to the "other doctors" in the medical profession to explicate by being placed on Axis III, then it is implied that there is no somatoform interest in the case. If the presentation is physical, the psychological need not be considered a factor in the presentation itself. If it is psychological, then the physical aspects of this syndrome can be avoided, diminished, or simply discounted. One is not allowed to have it both ways. It is a pressing question as to why the design of DSM-IV does not allow it both ways. The unsatisfactory nature of DSM-IV becomes clearer and the diagnostic process becomes more frustrating. Each diagnosis insists on exclusory criteria to eliminate the other diagnoses. The maze of uncertainty mounts. Here is the conundrum. Why can one not diagnose the patient as suffering from intertwined psychological and physical factors?[72]

The complexity of somatic syndromes in contrast to the relatively clear-cut and identifiable diagnostic categories of the DSM creates a profound difficulty for clinicians in the field. Martin's solution is to propose an alternative classification of somatoform disorders that divides these conditions into external disorders, in which the environment works upon a susceptible individual, and internal disorders, in which there is no immediate environmental influence.[73] External disorders are stress induced and internal ones are not. He further divides external disorders into three subclasses: acute, chronic, and psychiatric disorders that lead through body interaction to physical illness. Acute disorders include somatization disorders (due to acute, stressful social situations), acute insomnias and traumas, and direct stimuli causing distress (electric shock, etc.).[74] Chronic disorders include somatization disorders that are stress induced over time and may include such problems as fibromyalgia and chronic fatigue syndrome, as well as chronic insomnias. Psychiatric disorders concern the physical pain associated with depressive disorders, anxiety disorders with physical complaints, hyperarousal states, pain disorders, and the like. Internal disorders include somatization disorders (physical symptoms used in place of emotional ones), conversion disorders, hypochondriasis, self-induced illness (e.g., suicide attempts with physical injuries), and the like.

This subclass also includes conditions such as Body Dysmorphic Disorder and disorders in which minor physical symptoms are misinterpreted in such a way as to suggest major physical disorders (e.g., dizziness suggesting brain tumor).[75] As a consequence of this arrangement, Martin argues that medical diseases are recognized as potentially genuine psychosomatic disorders.[76] The beauty of Martin's approach lies in his attempt to integrate description and causality and we believe he is correct in his assessment that, with psychosomatic illness, things are not always as simple as they may seem.

Martin is not alone in his suggestion that current thinking about somatization often creates more problems than it solves. Sharpe and Carson address the issue of unexplained symptoms in the context of functional somatic syndromes and argue there is a need for a paradigm shift to make better sense of things. Functional somatic syndromes are made up of combinations of unexplained symptoms and, although "the research literature suggests the presence of biochemical and physiologic abnormalities in many of these disorders, they share a lack of the pathologically defined changes in tissue that designate medical conditions."[77] Examples of these syndromes include fibromyalgia, irritable bowel syndrome, and chronic fatigue syndrome. Historically, "unexplained symptoms" are those that remain after disease has been excluded and, the truth is, some symptoms which were previously regarded as unexplained, become explained when a cause is determined.[78] At the same time, there are occasions when new evidence has rendered symptoms previously considered explained to become unexplained, as is the case of chronic Epstein-Barr infection having been discredited as the explanation for most cases of chronic fatigue syndrome.[79] What is especially intriguing about Sharpe and Carson's paper is the attention they pay to much older notions about unexplained symptoms. At the end of the nineteenth century, the "accepted etiology of unexplained symptoms was a reversible functional disturbance of the nervous system, and the accepted treatment included attention to psychological aspects of medical management."[80] Interestingly, for treatment to be effective, it was considered important for it to be delivered in such a way that was congruent with patients' somatic view of their illness.[81] This look back is more than historical curiosity; Sharpe and Carson argue that much can be learned from the way unexplained symptoms were diagnosed and managed at that time.

> The predominant model was the functional nervous paradigm. This model explicitly acknowledged the neurobiological correlates of the patients' somatic symptoms as well as the influence of psychological factors. Symptoms were seen as a manifestation of a reversible functional disturbance rather than as fixed pathology of a purely psychological nature. Recent evidence has begun to provide support for this viewpoint. Endocrine and functional neurologic

as well as psychological factors are being identified in relation to functional syndromes. Examples include the irritable bowel syndrome, chronic pain and fatigue, repetitive strain injury, and even the archetypal psychogenic condition called conversion hysteria. Therefore, in part, patients may be correct that their symptoms are physical.[82]

The paradigm shift that Sharpe and Carson propose involves providing treatment in the context of medical consultation, thus viewing psychological and psychiatric interventions as integral to, rather than distinct from, the delivery of medical care. Furthermore, they insist that attention be paid to the psychological impact of the way in which symptoms are explained to patients and the use of psychotherapeutic techniques to facilitate a better doctor-patient relationship.[83]

The question remains whether Tsuang's use of the term "schizotaxia" might suggest an alternative way of thinking about somatoform disorders. What if we conceive of somatization as the prodromal phase which may or may not, under the right combination of circumstances, go on to manifest itself as hypochondriasis, and so forth? The idea is intriguing. While Somatization Disorder, Undifferentiated Somatoform Disorder, and Somatoform Disorder NOS, would indicate varying degrees of fully diagnostic somatization, Hypochondriasis, Body Dysmorphic Disorder, Pain Disorder, and Conversion Disorder would represent alternate pathways of expression. No doubt, the specific pathway would depend on neurobiological factors that are beyond the scope of this discussion. But, an approach such as this would point to the process of somatization as etiologically significant for all the somatoform disorders. The most obvious difficulty with this is the fact that not all of the somatoform disorders are functionally similar. Hypochondriasis relates to illness phobia and can be understood as ego-dystonic or ego-alien; the belief that the hypochondriac must have some kind of illness tends to be a source of unwelcome distress. Individuals with a somatization syndrome tend to present with genuine symptoms, even though the actual illness may lack biological markers. In contrast to the hypochondriac, the somatizer's condition tends to be ego-syntonic and more acceptable to the individual's sense of self, despite the fact that the symptoms themselves may be quite uncomfortable. Body Dysmorphic Disorder relates to self-perception and seems to involve something more akin to a body delusion than the displacement of psychological stress onto the body. Conversion symptoms also tend to be ego-dystonic and may resolve fairly rapidly, unlike the symptoms of somatization. These disorders possess apparent similarity by virtue of the fact that all of them directly involve a somatic focus; their functional dissimilarities, however, render it unlikely that all of them represent variants or subcategories of somatization. Reliance upon the DSM alone for an understanding of the process of somatization is problematic at best.

In addition, the existence of functional somatic syndromes introduces a diagnostic dilemma that the DSM seems unable to manage adequately. Somatization is a far more extensive and complex condition than the DSM Somatoform Disorders classification would lead one to believe. We understand the clinical exigencies which require a diagnosis in order to receive payment, and, the fact is, the clinician may be forced by practical necessity to resort to Undifferentiated Somatoform Disorder or Somatoform Disorder NOS to satisfy a managed care provider. But the patient with chronic pelvic pain or reflex sympathetic dystrophy, for example, is another matter. The day may well come when we look back and wonder how we ever imagined somatization to be a factor in these diagnoses. At the present, however, this is not the case and perpetuating the mind-body split by assuming these patients must have a DSM diagnosis and referring them to a behavioral health practitioner is not the magic bullet. For one thing, the psychiatrist will examine the medical record, note the predominance of a physiological condition, and, in the absence of clear psychiatric symptomology, may end up returning the patient to the referring physician. We give lip service to the idea of a mind-body interface, but we practice medicine as though it does not exist. Conventional thinking does not readily permit a great many options.

SOMATIZATION AS A PROCESS

We believe there is another, more viable approach to the situation. Martin, Robbins, and Kirmayer, and others are correct in thinking our understanding of somatization deepens when dimensional approaches are utilized in addition to the familiar descriptive ones of the DSM. However, we also believe somatization should be understood as a process that manifests itself not only in the symptoms that lend themselves to DSM classification, but also functional somatic syndromes that do not seem to lend themselves so easily to DSM categorization. As a process, somatization is far more complex than the diagnostic phenomenon with which most clinicians are familiar.

Nevertheless, diagnosis lies at the core of the medical model of psychological pathology and the diagnostic classification of disease is crucial. An adequate diagnostic system should not be restricted to description, but include the predictive and, hopefully, the prescriptive. Our task is to move beyond the conventional wisdom of observation alone to the study of causation. The core issue we need to address is the process of somatization itself.

Our premise is, when studying somatization as a process we need to begin with a framework that is broad enough to encompass the field. We begin by identifying the affected populations as chronic and situational subtypes.

While these are similar in some respects, they also differ. Somatization is an ego problem and chronic somatizers particularly suffer an ego-integrative defect. This means they experience impairment in executive functioning as it relates to problem solving, communication of emotions (alexithymia), or bodily sensations. The chronic subtype uses somatization to shore up ego functioning and, thus, symptom complaints are ego-syntonic and illness becomes a way of life. This patient tends to be the most treatment-resistant and is usually the one who comes most readily to mind when the term somatization is used in clinical contexts. Situational somatization (Situational Somatization Syndrome®) refers to those individuals who are prone to somatize in response to life stressors of the existential type. Generally more functional than the chronic subtype, situational somatizers are often overlooked by clinicians because their typical presentation is not suggestive of psychosomatic illness. As a result, treatment outcomes tend to be complicated and unsatisfactory.

Once we have identified the affected populations, we need to ask what characterizes their pathology across individual patient lines. Several issues require our attention at this point. Somatizing patients show a high degree of both interpersonal and intrapersonal ambivalence as well as a proclivity for progressive disorganization. Somatization is a defensive strategy that protects the fragile ego and creates a façade of normality. On the surface, these patients appear well organized but under stress, particularly interpersonal stress, they deteriorate and somatization becomes more pronounced.

As an aside, it is worth noting that ambivalence is observed among clinicians as well as patients. But clinician ambivalence is related to the mind-body interface and patient management. Somatization is possible because mind and body are codetermining in human experience. Traditional medical training, however, prepares us to regard mind and body separately. Only recently have programs in integrative medicine undergone development in major medical centers. It is very easy to look upon mind-body interactions as a New Age phenomenon. Clinicians can feel genuine ambivalence about the scientific validity of the concept. In addition, working with somatizing patients can generate enough drain on clinical resources to leave the physician feeling reticent about managing them in his or her practice. When we talk about causation in somatization, clinician ambivalence is a contributive factor that cannot be overlooked.

Somatizing patients are also relatively predisposed to difficulties integrating appearance and interpretation in perception. Perception is both conscious and unconscious. Somatizers present with diffuse pain and malaise reflecting disturbances in perception that can be traced to similar disturbances in psychological processing. Diminished ego capability results in a perceptual error whereby disturbances in psychological processing are interpreted as bodily symptoms. Multilevel perceptual diagnosis can be conducted empirically to specifically identify somatizing patients and testing development and procedures should be clarified.

The next step involves evaluating the intrapersonal structure that characterizes vulnerable members of somatizing populations. Generalized traits characterize a population but specific ones can be noted at the individual level. We employ the interpersonal theory of personality to identify patients at risk and show how somatization functions within four personality types. Impasse resistance can be resolved through an understanding of personality dynamics in somatization. In addition, warning signs for treatment failure, such as prepsychotic tendencies and paranoia, can be foreseen and strategies developed for their management.

When we have clarified the traits that characterize the somatizing populations as well as individuals within them, we are ready to discuss treatment. We discuss behavioral therapies and psychopharmacology in detail with respect to the chronic subtype. Because the ego-integrative defect can be quite profound in this group, therapy is directed toward symptom management. The resolution of somatization requires a degree of ego functioning that most chronic somatizers never develop for reasons related to genetics, family upbringing, and long-term use of somatization. In the absence of somatization, these patients frequently decompensate. Situational somatizers not only appear better organized, they also show some capability to tolerate more intensive therapies. Nevertheless, because their illness complaints are also defensive in nature, rather than confront them directly, we describe the use of short-term existential psychotherapy to address the existential crisis that necessitates somatization. Since we are dealing with poor ego integration that is present in varying degrees in these subtypes, clinician and treatment options take on the role of an auxiliary ego. The difficulty is we have to spend time with these patients in order to familiarize ourselves with their value system in order to provide the kind of executive functioning that will help them move in the direction they wish to go. Approaching treatment in the context of traits associated with the population and with the individual permits the tailoring of treatment to meet individual patient needs.

By approaching somatization from a process perspective, we circumvent the dilemma posed by diagnostic categories in favor of highlighting its underlying pathology. Ultimately, however we approach somatization, there is the danger that we may become so preoccupied with secondary phenomena that we neglect the primary one. We treat symptoms or functional somatic syndromes in the mistaken belief that these represent the essence of the patient's illness. In point of fact, they are the tip of the iceberg. If we are going to work with these patients effectively, we have to look beneath the surface where the bulk of their pathology is found. We must examine how somatization shores up ego functioning and select treatments that have a chance of success because they operate within the range of a patient's capability. By transcending our own limitations, we learn how to provide better care for our patients.

Chapter Two

Somatization and Its Discontents

Somatization is problematic for everyone involved in the delivery of health care services. Patient, provider, and third-party payer frequently feel uneasy, restless, deprived, frustrated, or ineffectual, all in turn. To begin with, the patient trusts the clinician to identify the disease that lies at the root of their symptoms and then design a plan which focuses not only on symptom alleviation but also disease elimination. If the clinician alludes to the presence of psychological factors, the patient typically regards this as evidence of the clinician's incompetence or, at best, inexperience. Discontent with the clinician, the patient seeks treatment elsewhere. Even in those cases where the clinician resists mentioning psychology, there is the difficulty of obtaining authorization for ongoing care. Insurance case managers are frequently discontented with patients who seem to require an inordinate amount of financial resources for treatment-intractable conditions.

It has been said, tongue in cheek, that the word "time" is perhaps one of the most feared and hated words in the English language. It makes an appearance late at night in every British pub, at that judicious or injudicious moment when the familiar, yet dreadful, message is announced during the last round, "Time, gentlemen, please!" Time is a precious commodity for patient, provider, and payer. The patient wants more time from the provider, but the provider can't exceed the time allowed by the payer, whose diagnosis related group (DRG) establishes the parameters for time-to-treat for a given condition. And the treatment of somatization demands time, usually much more than seems appropriate, and, as we all know, time is money.

In any case, the patient is miserable; the provider may not fully understand the mind-body interface sufficiently to communicate it with either patients or third-party payers who are themselves confused as to how or what to underwrite in order to compensate the provider for services within their often rigid system time frame. As a result, the provider is sandwiched in the middle between patients who feel lost in the shuffle and the payer knows little or nothing about the objective parameters surrounding the somatization problem. The provider, who is expected to understand the dynamics of somatization, lacks sufficient insight into the underlying psychopathology within the mind-body interface to provide necessary solutions for the payer to actuate. How did we arrive at this unfortunate state of affairs?

When Stekel coined the term "somatization," it's doubtful he had any idea where his semantics would lead. In the famous Dora case, Freud used hypnosis to cure his patient's neurosis and, by extension, provided alleviation for her physical symptoms. This, of course, led to the idea that somehow physical symptoms and psychological neuroses were intertwined. For many years, this held sway in psychiatric circles. However, with the advent of biological treatments for severe psychiatric illnesses, the focus began to shift from mind-body interactions to neurobiological causation. As will be discussed further in the next chapter, this shift represented a theoretical orientation based on the notion that mind and body were distinct, rather than interdependent, entities. To a certain extent, this makes sense. If you have a pharmacological agent that reduces symptoms, it's logical to assume it has a biological basis. The next step is to presume psychological influences are epiphenomenal rather than etiological.

But what if that's not the case? What if your patient's symptoms are genuinely biological and respond to biological treatments, but stem from a psychological influence? As long as the clinician is convinced that physical disease has to have a strictly biological basis, psychological factors will be excluded. The result of poor treatment outcomes is the kind of discontent we described in the beginning of this chapter. We need to become more adaptable in our thinking. Osteopathic physicians have long held that the term "illness" represents the disease plus the patient. This means we can't isolate the disease from the patient's experience and perceptions and that brings us back to our original contention, that is, somatization is not simply a diagnostic category but an illness condition that is indistinguishable from patients themselves. In our discussions of causality, we have to examine the patient to see where somatic displacement comes from and how it functions.

While dimensional theories of psychopathology encourage us to think in terms of causality, little has actually been written on the personality factors involved in the process of somatization. Barsky argues that some patients are fearful of pain and become anxious when faced with the prospect of experiencing discomfort. These individuals can be called *amplifiers* and anxiety intensifies or "amplifies" their experience of physical symptoms. Among these individuals, emotional and "bodily distress becomes a loop in which each form of suffering perpetuates and intensifies the other."[1] The inclination of amplifiers to consciously overestimate the significance of symptoms and the degree of harm they may experience is a primary factor that sets the somatization cycle in motion. Catastrophic thinking leads to hypervigilance and repetitive checking behaviors as well as the need for reassurance.[2] Barsky's idea would likely be well accepted among cognitive behaviorists who are accustomed to tracing distress responses to faulty or irrational beliefs.

Hamlin has researched the role of psychological problems in successful surgical outcomes directed at pain relief.[3] The focus of his investigation was the evaluation of a new instrument for personality assessment developed by the senior author for identifying and quantifying factors that correlated with poor surgical outcomes and to assess the specificity and predictive power of the test algorithm in patients undergoing laminectomy and carpal-tunnel surgery. Increased somatic symptom fixation was observed relative to significant elevation in repression and suggestibility, depression, compulsive personality defense features, social/cultural defensiveness, low ego functions, and low self-esteem, all of which correlated with somatic displacement. Of those patients demonstrating the somatization process in the Hamlin study, three variations of personality profiles were noted: (1) the depressed compulsive patient with high somatic complaints, (2) the dependent, love-oriented, fearful, labile patient with bodily symptom focus, and (3) the depressed, fearful, phobic-type patient with anxiety expressed in the form of body phobia rather than patients with phobias of external objects.[4] Analysis of the Hamlin study data revealed that not only did those patients with poor surgical outcomes tend to be somatizers, but most chronic-type somatizers expressed conflict or ambivalence between their self-report and preconscious personality levels; nonsomatizers did not show these features.[5] These results are consistent with the internalizer (individuals sensitive to mismatch) as well as those patients prone to the amplification and prolongation of physical symptom complaints. In addition to the presenting evidence for somatization in test findings was the conspicuous absence of indicators for prior somatization in some patient clinical histories, a factor consistent with situational-type somatization.

The somatization process involves more than the psychological perception or misperception of sensations: it possesses a biophysical component as well. Sixty years ago we didn't talk about mental disorders in terms of neurotransmitters, genetic predispositions, and neuro-deficient circuits. Psychoanalytic doctrine, for example, regarded hypochondria as a somatic riddle that was part and parcel of dependency and low self-esteem. Clearly, the psychogenic tradition granted too much power to the workings of the human mind and fell short of acknowledging biological and cultural factors, patterns of family life, ethnicity, and gender.

We now know that effective chemical treatments suggest the presence of a biological component in the various mental disorders, and current evidence points to dysregulation in the serotonin system as one of the major players. Serotonin, which is plentiful in the limbic region of the brain, regulates emotion and seems to influence a number of bodily and mental processes, including mood, appetite, pain transmission, sleep, and sexual behavior. Current theory implicates downstream effects of serotonin reuptake inhibition at the cellular level in the development of mood disorders.[6] Impulsive behavior, such as aggression and suicide, seem to be influenced by the serotonin system, although the specific mechanisms involved are still unknown.

Eric Hollander sees a number of neurologically linked conditions resting along a continuum of what he calls, "obsessive-spectrum" disorders.[7] At one end, we find the compulsive or risk-aversive type disorders which are characterized by ruminative thoughts or preoccupation with physical defects, either real or imagined. For example, in Body Dysmorphic Disorder the patient's anxiety is focused on the body's appearance, in anorexia nervosa the anxiety is related to weight, and in hypochondriasis the anxiety is concerned with illness. Located at the other end of the continuum are the impulsive or risk-seeking disorders which are marked by ritual-driven behaviors such as hypersexuality or aggressive acting out often associated with high-adrenaline personalities.

There is evidence of an overlap between compulsive and impulsive symptomology both in families as well as individuals. While it is not unusual to see these behaviors expressed in clusters, generally speaking, the traits tend to remain isolated from one another. The impulsive types seeking high-stimulus behaviors and the compulsives rigidly stuck in harm-avoidance and fear. Another way of putting it is to view the impulsive individuals as "externalizers" and the compulsives as "internalizers." Those who are prone to exaggerate the possibility of harm associated with actions or thoughts tend to be hypervigilant and sensitive to subtle changes in sensory input. According to Hollander, there seems to be an internal alarm that goes off when something doesn't feel or look quite right.[8] This "alarm" functions as a kind of mismatch indicator. The "mismatch hypothesis," so to speak, is quite similar to Barsky's cognitive notion, but rather than blame bad habits or faulty learning, neurobiologists attribute the problem to a brain abnormality that causes persons to scan their environment with heightened sensitivity.

In addition to the psychological, biological, and genetic factors related to somatization, there are cultural ones. Social science has pointed out for some time that the experience of health and sickness goes beyond psyche and soma, and must be examined with the context of culture and the times in which we live. Symptoms have a social as well as individual stamp, according to Shorter, who argues there is something outside the self—social mores, marital dynamics, etc.—that direct behavior for dealing with emotions and illness. In our culture, hypochondriacal and somatic concerns cross the lines of gender, age, ethnic, and socioeconomic status. The expression of symptoms is often handled quite differently from one ethnic group to another. Persons from lower socioeconomic levels who report having less education tend to suffer more unexplained medical symptoms. The divorced, separated, widowed, or unmarried are at a greater risk for disease than those who are married. Persons over age 65 often experience chronic physical illness, but are less prone to hypochondriacal complaints than younger individuals. Somatic displacement and somatization tend to affect both genders equally, but women frequently suffer more vague physical ailments for which they seek medical attention than do men. Every generation has its own brand of vague physical complaints: Yesterday's neurasthenia has become today's fibromyalgia. It is clear we are dealing with a complex phenomenon when trying to unravel the contributing factors to the somatization process.

There is a long history in medicine in which somatizing syndromes have been understood and treated largely by attending to patients' physical symptom complaints. Over the latter part of the past century, however, the collective conscious awareness among catalogers has assigned a greater importance to clustering symptoms and assigning them to discrete disorders. What has yet to emerge is the idea that somatization is itself symptomatic of an actual mind-body interface. Poorly understood, unexplained, or subjectively expressed symptom complaints, which lack the tissue changes associated with physiological pathology, have become known in recipe cookbook terms as somatizing syndromes to the many medical specialties.

Somatizing conditions must fit the rules and norms currently used in the medical model, which tell us that a particular collection of symptom-based criteria has sufficient specificity, sensitivity, frequency, demonstrated usefulness, and plausibility, to qualify for a designation in the "disease" category. After all, there are no apparently explicit definitions of terms in use explaining which symptom clusters qualify for inclusion as a "disease" per se. Lines of demarcation separating the semantics of progression from sign to symptom, symptom to syndrome, and syndrome to disease are rather loose, if not entirely arbitrary. Biological and clinical considerations have been suggested to assist in establishing the boundaries among these terms, but society ultimately determines their utility, dictating where somatization falls within the disease continuum.

Considering the complexity of mind-body interface, we might offer some clarity by speaking in terms of "symptom becoming disease." Hence, the title of this book refers to patients in distress and who seek help from clinicians for their physical symptom complaints. Symptoms are patients' expressions of the subjective experience of changes within their bodies. Diseases are objectively observed abnormalities which stem from the identification of physical causative factors. A different kind of disease is diagnosed when symptoms reflect the mind-body interface, and we call this somatization. In essence, when the clinician is unable to establish a pathologically defined physical disease as causative of the patient's symptoms, but *is* able to uncover the emotionally induced stress reactions of the patient which are somatically displaced, s/he is in the presence of somatization. The detection of this comorbid condition is made, either through the clinician's own sensitive perceptions of the patient or additionally through the use of a special test, such as the Paindex® Test, which is designed to establish the proclivity for somatization. After the diagnosis of a potential somatizing syndrome is entertained and before that diagnosis is established, the clinician must decide whether s/he wants to follow this patient. Any treatment plan must be seriously thought out before one commits to the often lengthy supportive therapeutic relationship necessary to mutually explore the meaning of the patient's symptoms. The treatment plan is where the real difficulties are first encountered, where the seeds of discontent are often planted.

The resistance to admitting a psychological element in physical symptoms is counterbalanced by an opposite tendency observed in some individuals; that is, a resistance to reporting pain and/or other physical symptoms. We are all familiar with athletes who "play hurt," and seem capable of rather heroic performance despite obvious injury. To some extent, however, this notion may represent something of an urban myth. At least one author has drawn attention to the questionable practice of administering local anesthetic injections to enable football and rugby players to engage in play without pain.[9] Nevertheless, sports literature is replete with accounts of cyclists, long distance runners, and others, who are able to transcend pain by training, endurance, and the drive to win. It is a different matter with individuals who suffer from anosognosia; that is, the failure to acknowledge, or be distressed by, one's physical disability. Anosognosia has been studied in a variety of patients including those with phantom limb syndrome, hemiplegia, and schizophrenia.[10] As such, it does not seem to be a condition that we can easily attribute to individuals who are disinclined to report physical symptoms. The clinical literature has not devoted a great deal of attention to these individuals, so we are left somewhat to our own devices.

Considerable attention has been given, however, to pain tolerance and here we might gain some insight. Studies indicate several factors are involved in pain tolerance. In a study of chronic pain sufferers, Edwards et al. determined that white patients tend to have greater pain tolerance than African Americans over a broad range of age and populations.[11] Examining individual pain history and familial pain tolerance models in post-surgical pain, Bachiocco et al. found that individuals with a previous pain history as well as poor familial pain tolerance tended to experience earlier and more severe post-surgical pain.[12] In a study of male and female subjects with Temperomandibular Disorder, Bragdon et al. suggest differing physiological analgesic mechanisms may be implicated in pain response.[13] Studying affective processing and attention, de Wied and Verbaten found priming and appraisal may be factors in pain tolerance.[14] When patients exposed to cold pressor pain were also exposed to unpleasant pictures that included pain-related material, it was observed they tolerated the cold water for shorter periods than did those subjects whose pictures did not include pain-related material. The writers suggest that the presence and type of affective distractors may be meaningful for enhancing pain tolerance.[15] If we may abstract from increased pain tolerance, we might assume these individuals also tend to either underreport or, at least, less frequently report, the experience of physical pain.

In addition to ethnicity, gender, and biological factors, there may be other considerations involved among individuals who are resistant to reporting symptoms. For example, there are those persons who seem eager to be perceived as "good patients." These individuals often seem very concerned about how the doctor is feeling, whether s/he is tired or busy, and they minimize their own complaints in comparison. In such cases, underreporting symptoms functions in a defensive manner to ward off anxiety associated with concerns the patient has about disappointing the doctor, or perhaps of having a more serious condition than has been diagnosed. Family pressures to be "strong" or cultural stereotypes that reward the athlete who continues to play despite obvious injury may also function in the resistance to downplay symptom severity. In chapter 7 of this volume, the authors discuss personality factors that seem to figure strongly in those individuals with somatization. One might be tempted to presume that so-called symptom-tolerant individuals possess opposite personality characteristics. While this remains to be seen, we know that not all those with what we might call "vulnerable" personality types utilize somatization. As a consequence, it seems unlikely that we can draw a simple correlation between personality type alone and symptom resistance.

If we regard somatization as the preoccupation with physical symptoms, do we describe those who resist reporting symptoms as nonsomatizers? If that is the case, then how do we define the vast majority of patients who are simply concerned with how they feel? There seems to be a qualitative difference between those who minimize symptoms for whatever reason and those who are neither predisposed to preoccupation with symptoms or the minimization of symptoms. Accordingly, underreporting of symptom severity is a far more complex matter than simply disease preoccupation or its absence. One thing does seem reasonably clear: a reverse process is involved. For the somatizer, the body carries the burden of psychological conflict. Among those who underreport pain, the mind seems to act as a buffer, literally diminishing the awareness of illness or transforming it into a meaningful experience that reinforces ego strength. While the somatizing patient views pain as evidence of some physical malady, the pain-tolerant individual seems to regard this experience as evidence of personal durability.

In any case, the fact remains that some individuals proceed from physical pain toward psychological resilience while others proceed from psychological vulnerability toward physical illness. While the mind-body interface enables the process of somatization in a top-down fashion, it also seems to work to produce greater tolerance of physical symptoms in those individuals so predisposed. Admittedly, the focus of the current work is on the patient who relies on physical illness to express psychological conflict, but the idea of deriving critical information about one condition by studying its opposite is not new. In recent years, researchers have given increased attention to individuals who demonstrate resiliency in the face of trauma in the hope of nurturing similar qualities in those who have been disabled by traumatic life events. Similarly, we suspect research into the behavior and personality traits of persons who seem symptom-resilient, as well as the potentially adaptive functions of these characteristics, might lead to a greater understanding of the ways we might engender similar traits in those who are prone to somatization.

Somatization is a complex of psychological, biological, social, and cultural factors that may render patient evaluation, treatment, and payment for services problematic. Clinicians, patients, and insurance carriers are all ambivalent and for their own reasons. As the wise sage points out, sometimes the only way out of a dilemma is through it and that is certainly the case with ambivalence. It is to this, we now turn.

Chapter Three

A View from Outside the Box

When asked what they like about their doctor patients usually mention something about a "good bedside manner." They go on to say s/he is patient and a good listener, seems interested in what they have to say, and makes them feel like s/he cares. In short, patients are describing the clinician's ability to convey a sense of empathy. Carl Rogers, the psychologist who developed the Person-Centered Approach to psychotherapy, insisted the therapist had to communicate unconditional positive regard for the patient.[1] The clinician should be accepting, nonjudgmental, and make an effort to genuinely understand patients and why they behave as they do. With some, this is easy: The patient has an interesting history, is motivated to improve, and is pleasant and engaging. With somatizing patients, however, it is not so simple. Diagnostic uncertainty, time constraints, the perception that this represents a "difficult" population, and minimal training in behavioral medicine are among the factors that contribute to clinicians feeling ambivalent about somatizing patients.[2] In some cases, even more intense feelings, including anger and resentment, may surface as the result of a poor treatment alliance.

While ambivalence is natural given the ambiguous nature of relating to somatizers, it can exert a detrimental effect on patient care, particularly when it goes unrecognized. As we shall discuss in later chapters, ambivalence and difficulty identifying emotions are characteristic of somatizing patients. Emotional self-awareness is a very beneficial tool for the practicing clinician.[3] More than self-awareness is required, however, when addressing ambivalence because it tends to be rooted, at least in part, in our training and, as a result, it can be ubiquitous in the encounter with somatizing patients. In order to create meaningful therapeutic relationships, it is critical that clinicians be well acquainted with their own ambivalence, its sources, and its resolution.

To begin with, insofar as our current system of graduate psychological and medical education can be understood to be based on the scientific method, we can say that, to a certain extent, it actually fosters ambivalence. The scientific method is based on the principle that an ontological distinction exists between an object of inquiry and an observing subject. In other words, in the very nature of the case, subject and object are absolutely separate entities. In truth, it seems necessary to have such a distinction in order to engage in the process of observation, experimentation, measurement, and analysis. If the subject and object are not distinct from one another, how can we know with any assurance that our observations are objective? This was, essentially, the dilemma faced by the philosopher Rene Descartes, whose work provides the basis for much of our modern thinking in this regard.

Descartes is probably most remembered for his famous maxim, cogito ergo sum—I think, therefore I am.[4] At first blush, it sounds like Descartes was struggling with the question of his own existence, and in fact, that's not far off the mark. Cogito ergo sum represents Descartes' attempt to establish the possibility of knowing that the universe possesses an actual physical reality and is not merely the product of a mental illusion or fantasy. Descartes began with the premise that he would exclude from philosophical speculation anything about which doubt could be entertained. In so doing, he came to the realization that the one thing he absolutely could not doubt was the fact that he "doubted" at all. The reality of his own ability to think and use doubt as a rational process indicated that he, himself, must exist—and his mind as an entity distinct from his body. "From that I knew that I was a substance the whole essence or nature of which is to think, and that for its existence there is no need of any place, nor does it depend on any material thing; so that this 'me,' that is to say, the soul by which I am what I am, is entirely distinct from body, and is even more easy to know than the latter; an even if body were not, the soul would not cease to be what it is."[5] Utilizing his own existence as an irreducible point of certitude, Descartes was able to establish what he regarded as a reliable knowledge about God and the physical world.[6]

The effect of Cartesian dualism on the scientific method stems from the philosophical position that mind and body are distinct entities. It follows that one should be able to "stand outside" an object of inquiry with the result that one's observations possess the quality of objectivity. The importance of this presupposition cannot be underestimated. The proposition that mind and body are profoundly separate leads to the conclusion that an object can be studied in situ and remain unchanged. While this is a worthy goal, it has received considerable criticism in such fields as anthropology where it is generally regarded as impossible to observe an indigenous culture without, in fact, altering the culture itself.

More to the point of our discussion, in the field of psychotherapy the possibility of an objective analyst or therapist has received quite a bit of attention. One of the hallmarks of Sigmund Freud's practice of psychoanalysis was his insistence that the analyst sit behind patients, outside their field of vision, so as to avoid contaminating the patient's free associations. The idea was the analyst presented a "blank screen" upon which the patients could project their psychic contents and relive past behavior patterns in a transference relationship with the analyst. In this way, the patient might experience the analyst as the "rejecting parent," for example, and come to some resolution of neurotic conflicts. Freud was quite insistent that psychoanalysis required analytic objectivity; without it, analysis was impossible. Ideas change over time and Freud's position has come under attack by non-psychoanalytic writers as well as Neo-Freudians such as Otto Rennick and Thomas Ogden.[7]

Glen O. Gabbard, MD, notes that a "burgeoning literature on social constructivism, mutuality, intersubjectivity, relativism, and perspectivism has stressed that absolute objectivity is a myth and that the analyst's subjectivity inevitably enters into perceptions of the analysand."[8] While he is reticent about abandoning the field entirely to post-modernism which argues that objectivity is, prima face, impossible, Gabbard reminds us that our own subjective experience of patients (countertransference) gives us vital information about their condition, emotional state, beliefs, and so forth that we dare not neglect. Gabbard concludes:

> An analyst who sees the database as the patient's subjective experience, while treating his or her countertransference experiences as only interferences or obstacles, is depriving the patient of an important developmental experience... Hence providing a different perspective, that of the subjectivity of the analyst, in contrast to trying simply to locate the patient's perspective, is a critically important aspect of the analyst's functioning. In this regard the analyst is objective in the sense that he or she is an object external to the thinking mind of the patient.[9]

In simpler terms, therapy or analysis is incomplete unless we recognize that the subjective experiences of both patient and therapist are profoundly connected in the same dynamic relationship. We believe the arguments presented concerning the analyst's objectivity and subjectivity hold true for both medical and psychological clinicians.

Granted, the conditions involved in a medical examination seem rather different from those encountered in psychotherapy, although it can be argued rather cogently that it's not all that different, and the establishment of a relationship based on trust is critical for a positive outcome to medical treatment. Nevertheless, we are trained in medical school and residency to distance ourselves, to a certain extent, from patient distress so that we can treat disease effectively. There is no question that clinical practice requires at least some emotional distance on the part of the physician. Indeed, even the practiced psychotherapist must limit the extent to which s/he is affected or, perhaps, infected, by a patient's distress in order to be effective as a clinician. As Gabbard has wisely noted, we must be able to speak to a patient's needs from our own point of view: "The presence of the analyst's subjectivity does not automatically eliminate the validity of that analyst's outside or object-based perception."[10]

Part and parcel of our subjective experience of the patient is our conviction that we have something useful to impart to the patient based on reasonable evidence. However, simply because we are working with physical illness does not preclude the fact that we are primarily working with persons. And whenever we are involved with persons, relationships become a factor and this is where things may become complicated.

Because we are involved with the patient as a real person, there is the potential for ambivalence to factor into the relationship. A patient-centered approach to health care reminds us that, while illness may deprive an individual of health, it does not deprive them of humanity. Wise teachers remind student doctors that, ultimately, their patients are persons who need to be attended with respect and a willingness to listen. In a real sense, the doctor-patient relationship is pregnant with possibilities: We influence the patient and the patient influences us in a dynamic that precludes absolute objectivity. When patients enter the examination room, they may feel vulnerable, uncertain, and even fearful. We respond with knowledge, confidence, and hope—all factors which take us beyond the boundaries of objective reality and thrust us into subjectivity. In order to allay patients' fears we become human. We may lay an assuring hand on a shoulder, we soften our tone of voice, our eyes convey compassion, and we ourselves become vulnerable in that moment. This can be unnerving, especially for the student doctor or psychology intern who naturally feels the anxiety that accompanies inexperience. Clinicians need to be mindful that close association with persons in distress will not only remind them of their own susceptibility to pain and illness but also of the impossibility of being completely emotionally disengaged with patients and their suffering.

Magnify the intensity of working with ordinary patients several fold, and the degree of ambivalence one experiences when working with a resistant population becomes more easily recognizable. Coping with the whole complex of symptom complaints, failed treatments, repeated referrals, and uncertain etiologies may leave the physician feeling as though s/he is locked in an endless struggle with the Tar Baby of the Uncle Remus stories. As the reader will surely recall, Tar Baby was a figure created out of tar by a wily fox and bear who sought to entrap Br'r Rabbit for their supper. As the story unfolds, Br'r Rabbit tries to engage Tar Baby in ordinary chit chat; when Tar Baby remains silent, Br'r Rabbit assumes he has been insulted. He strikes Tar Baby with one paw, then another, and soon all four paws are trapped. The more Br'r Rabbit struggled, the more he seemed unable to free himself. Ethically and professionally motivated to provide quality care, the clinician becomes ensnared in what appears as the patient's treatment resistance.

Consider the following case in point. A young woman with cerebral palsy was undergoing psychiatric treatment for symptoms of Bulimia. She reports that, over the past year, she has been neither eating nor drinking consistently, but shows no signs of weight loss or dehydration. Recently, the patient's mother discovered she had resumed her binge-purge behavior, and as part of their agreement, she had been told to leave the house (the daughter was allowed to live at home as long as she wasn't symptomatic). Over the course of the past few months, the patient has developed frequent urinary tract infections and has become intolerant of oral antibiotics. Since leaving her mother's home, she developed mild pylonephritis and was hospitalized for treatment with IV antibiotics. On the date of her discharge, she returned later to the ER complaining of severe abdominal pain. With her therapist and psychiatrist she now presents as severely regressed, focusing solely on her somatic symptoms, and unable to talk through such psychological issues as her relationship with her mother. Frustrated with the patient's resistance and ambivalent about continuing to work with her, psychiatrist and therapist, as well as the patient's family physician, have discussed transferring her to other providers. There are times when the clinician wonders whether s/he has decidedly correctly about treatment or whether someone else might be a better fit for a particular patient. These are the normal concerns one entertains when evaluating patient resistance. Ambivalence enters the picture when the clinician is undecided, when s/he teeters between the desire to prescribe treatment, and the wish to be someplace else.

Clinician ambivalence is all the more predictable when one neglects to take into account the mind-body interface. As long as physical symptoms are regarded as the evidence of physical illness alone, a wider range of diagnostic considerations is excluded. For a number of very good reasons, clinicians may be reticent about including psychosomatics in the differential diagnosis of physical symptomology. Liability and the desire to provide meaningful medical care are two examples. There may also be genuine uncertainty as to the validity of the mind-body concept and its effect on symptom generation. In the latter case, medical science itself comes to the rescue and provides evidence of its own that things are not always as they seem.

We are all familiar with the double-blind placebo-controlled study which serves as the "gold standard" for pharmacological testing. The efficacy of a pharmacological agent is measured against the use of an inert or inactive substance which serves as an experimental control. Interestingly enough, in most experiments one observes a certain percent of tested individuals who respond to placebo as though it had some treatment efficacy. Typically, we tend to presume placebo responders suffer from hypochondriasis or some other disingenuous condition which predisposes them to respond positively to any agent. In some cases, there is actually a relatively small difference between the numbers of drug and placebo responders. Particularly, relative to antidepressant medication trials, some researchers have recently suggested that this factor indicates that antidepressant medications are not as effective as we have been led to believe.[11] One wonders, however, if there are not specific characteristics which determine whether a placebo response will take place and, if so, might this indicate conditions under which a placebo might actually have some serious medical application? This is precisely the argument put forth by Walter A. Brown, MD, of Brown University School of Medicine.[12]

Over the past several years, Brown and his colleagues have gathered considerable data concerning the nature of placebo responders in antidepressant drug trials.[13] Specifically, antidepressant improvement with placebo is associated with a relatively short depressive illness, evidence of a precipitating event, depression of moderate global severity, and a good response to previous antidepressant treatment.[14] In short, at least where depressed patients are concerned, placebo responders are not necessarily the anomalous population we have heretofore assumed them to be. Instead, they possess specific characteristics that render them good prospects for a trial of placebo antidepressant treatment. But placebos aren't restricted to psychiatric treatment; quite to the contrary, they have demonstrated efficacy in the treatment of strictly medical conditions such as tissue damage and post-surgical pain.[15]

There are other factors, however, involved in generating a valid placebo response besides the administration of an injection or the taking of a pill. A meaningful and effective relationship with patients is a vital element and includes such factors as an expert healer, a thorough evaluation coupled with an explanation for the patient's distress, expectation of improvement, the clinician's commitment, enthusiasm and positive regard, the opportunity for the patient to verbalize distress, and a plausible treatment.[16] It is noteworthy that we frequently assume these elements are essential to the ways we interact with patients; in that sense, we may endorse the placebo effect without even knowing it.

Ultimately, the importance of the placebo effect lies in the fact that it affirms the presence of a mind-body interface. If placebo responders could be dismissed simply as individuals who were very susceptible to suggestion, we could stop right here. But the research of Brown et al. is compelling: Under certain conditions, the administration of an inert substance is sufficient to activate neurochemical processes with the result that symptom reduction takes place. The information-processing and integrative functions of the cerebral cortex which we associate with the term "mind" exert a demonstrable effect on the "purely physiological mechanisms" of the body. For example, in a PET scan–based study of male patients with unipolar depression, administered placebo as part of an inpatient imaging study of fluoxetine, Mayberg et al. determined that "placebo response was associated with regional metabolic increases involving the prefrontal, anterior cingulate, premotor, parietal, posterior insula, and posterior cingulate and metabolic decreases involving the subgenual cingulate, parahippocampus, and thalamus . . . regions of change overlapped those seen in responders administered active fluoxetine."[17] It's true that fluoxetine response was associated with additional subcortical and limbic changes, but the point is, the placebo response was not only measurable, but affected the same regions as the active antidepressant.[18] If the mind can generate a positive physiologic response to a placebo, it stands to reason the mind can generate the symptoms which necessitate treatment in the first place.

This line of thinking has begun to receive more attention in the literature concerning the neurophysiologic effects of psychotherapy. In contrast to the tendency to divide mental disorders into psychological and biological categories, the former to be treated with psychotherapy and the latter with medication, there is growing interest in the idea that psychotherapy works, at least in part, by producing changes in neural structure and functioning. A key element in this line of thinking concerns the effects of an organism's environment on neural plasticity. Gabbard draws upon both animal and human models to demonstrate the effects of the environment on neural plasticity, for example the altering of synaptic connections and changes in neurotransmitter activity.[19] Schuessler points to the effects of the environment on gene expression.

> Environmental factors determine the expression of specific genes and in turn, the proteins produced change the environment so that new genes are expressed. Thus there develops a self-organizing process under the control of a continuous dialogue between the genome and the environment. This results increasingly in the formation of more and more complex structures. The additive model of "gene + environment = phenotype" must be given up and the answer to the question as to what determines behavior is not simply nature or nurture, but rather that nature and nurture interact.[20]

The interaction of nature and nurture is one way of conceptualizing psychotherapy. Whether we are using behavior therapy to produce extinction of anxiety-related responses, cognitive-behavior therapy to alter irrational thinking, or psychodynamic therapy to reprocess affect-laden experiences, therapy represents a significant environmental influence on the patient in terms of experiential learning and relearning.[21]

The effects of learning on neural plasticity have been the subject of a great deal of study. Donald Hebb, a pioneer in this area, postulated that neuronal cortical connections are strengthened and remodeled by experience, and he showed that rats that were allowed to run freely around his house were better learners and had better memory capacity than rats that were kept in the laboratory.[22]

In this regard, it has been noted that an activity-rich environment has a number of effects on the brain including increasing the number of neuronal connections, particularly in the somatic sensory system.[23] In the brains of musicians, long-term motor training and repeated practice of complicated bimanual motor activity leads to changes, both in brain structure and in representation of brain cortical motor maps.[24] Specifically, the anterior corpus collosum, which is composed of nerve fibers connecting the frontal motor-related regions and pre-frontal regions which are critical for coordination of bimanual motor activity, has been found to be larger in musicians that began musical training before age seven than in musicians who began their training later.[25]

Changes in brain structure have also been observed in psychotherapy studies. For example, there is evidence that behavior therapy for Obsessive-Compulsive Disorder produces changes in caudate nucleus function.[26] In a neuroimaging study of twenty-four depressed patients treated with paroxetine or Interpersonal Psychotherapy (IPT), Brody et al. found that in the IPT group, PET scans showed a highly significant increase in activity in the inferior frontal gyrus and anterior insula for all subjects.[27] In an MRI study of patients with spider phobia, Paquette et al observed activation of the right dorsolateral prefrontal cortex, parahippocampal gyrus, and visual associative cortical areas when patients were presented with film images of spiders.[28] Following a successful course of cognitive-behavioral therapy, no significant activation of the right dorsolateral prefrontal cortex and parahippocampal gyrus was observed, leading the authors to observe that changes made at the level of the mind, within a psychotherapeutic context, are able to functionally "rewire" the brain.[29] A recent MEDLINE study by Roffman indicates initial neuroimaging studies have revealed convergent and mechanistically sensible effects of psychotherapy on brain function across a range of psychiatric disorders.[30] According to Liggan and Kay, an increase in the number and size of synapses depends on the region of the brain that is measured and the kind of therapy or differential experience the individual has undergone: "Whether the brain shows plastic changes in response to a particular kind of experience depends on the brain region, the kind of experience, and special circumstances or treatments that enhance or impair plasticity."[31] They go on to relate several psychotherapeutic models to those regions of the brain where we are likely to observe changes.

Behavioral psychotherapy focuses on dysfunction in simple forms of learning and memory (operant and associative conditioning) and related motor behavior. This paradigm involves brain structures such as the amygdala, basal ganglia, and hippocampus. Cognitive psychotherapy focuses on specific patterns of information processing. These symptoms are used as clues by which to define specific verbal thoughts and assumptions or schemata that account for both the symptomatic state and the psychological vulnerability to that state. Cognitive theory predicts the kinds of thinking patterns encountered with each disorder. Thus, the initial objectives of treatment are to teach the patient to recognize these cognitions. Thereafter, the patient learns to evaluate and modify such thinking patterns. Therapy then focuses on the identification and modification of dysfunctional attitudes that are inferred from the patient's stereotyped thinking and behavioral patterns. These schemata are values derived from early life experiences and support moment-to-moment thinking patterns. Putative brain areas include the neocortex, specifically the frontal cortex. Psychodynamic psychotherapy has as its central focus interpersonal representation: a set of expectations about self, others, and their relationship that organizes related affect, thought, and behavior. The neuropsychological underpinnings of interpersonal representations probably involve complex neurocircuitry incorporating lateralized cerebral hemispheres and subcortical areas.[32]

If environmental factors such as learning and psychotherapy have measurable effects on neurophysiology and, by implication, on gene expression, then we can no longer rely on Cartesian dualism to provide an adequate basis for thinking about mind and body. We are thrust by the evidence itself into the realm of the mind-body interface.

The overall intent of the present chapter has been, first of all, to help clear up any misconceptions the reader may have about the reality of the mind-body interface. Whether we are referring to the placebo effect or the impact of psychotherapy on neurobiology, we are really talking about the implications of measurable effects of psychological inputs on physiological outputs. Ultimately, this means we are going to deal with patients whose illness experience reflects a far more complicated and challenging clinical picture. This involves addressing our ambivalence as clinicians about mind-body illness and about the patients themselves.

We approach our uncertainty, doubt, and ambivalence about the role of the mind-body interface in somatic symptoms by study, evaluation of the available evidence, and consultation with peers. Over time we become more comfortable with illness conceptions that reflect a broader scientific base and our clinical practice follows accordingly. Gaining insight into one's sense of ambivalence about somatizing patients, however, is a more personal endeavor. At this point, clinicians must be willing to recognize that they have emotional responses to patients and some of these may seem less comfortable than others. We are all familiar with the satisfaction we experience with a patient who is motivated for treatment and puts forth tremendous effort to achieve symptom reduction. At the same time, there are other patients who generate more complicated emotions and leave us feeling baffled or frustrated. Personal communication with a number of clinicians has led the authors to believe that ambivalence is not only a painful experience for the clinician, but also has the potential to generate therapy-interfering behaviors on the part of the patient.

In the language of psychotherapy, we use the term "countertransference" to describe the clinician's feelings about the patient. To the extent we remain unaware of these feelings, we may unintentionally express them in ways that hinder the doctor-patient relationship. Patients are often notoriously adept at "reading" their doctor's emotional state, and comments such as "I think you must be tired of seeing me," or "I know you must have other more interesting patients to see," may be very accurate interpretations of our own ambivalence about the patient. True, comments such as these may be intended to elicit support from the clinician, reinforcement that we are indeed interested in their case and are committed to their care. But the underlying concern should not be ignored; communication takes place at multiple levels and verbal communication is only one of these.

In some cases, medical noncompliance, doctor shopping, body language, and so on can be understood to represent the patient's attempt to "act out" their sense of the clinician's ambivalence. By seeking another physician, they defend themselves against the anxiety they feel about being "too much trouble." We also need to be aware that patients may try to infuse us with their own ambivalence about their potential for treatment response. The technical term for this is "projection" and it describes the tendancy of patients to imagine that their own fears and hopelessness actually represent the experience of their clinician. What may be a difficult relationship in the first place is now more complicated by the patient's inability to tolerate the anxiety associated with their illness. In this way, the doubts entertained by the patient for their improvement are thrust upon the clinician. If we are not cautious, we will find ourselves colluding with the patient without even realizing it.

We want to make it clear that we don't expect the average primary care physician to undertake the process of personal analysis that is part and parcel of in-depth psychotherapy. What we wish to do is draw attention to is the need to become aware of the subtle ways we may influence patients by ignoring our own here and now feelings about them, including any sense of ambivalence we may experience about treating them in the first place. There is an old saying in psychotherapy: one cannot take a patient any further than one has gone oneself. Some would argue there are exceptions, and many times we see patients making gains which leave us in awe. For now, the point is, we can scarcely expect somatizing patients to manage their ambivalence about treatment, therapeutic intimacy, about establishing a lasting doctor-patient relationship, if we are not willing to take our feelings about them just as seriously.

Chapter Four

Ambivalence and Progressive Disorganization in Somatization

Clinician ambivalence is largely interpersonal and derives from real or potential interactions with patients. Ambivalence in somatization, however, incorporates both interpersonal and intrapersonal elements. Because of the presence of an "ego-integrative defect" that diminishes overall ego functioning, somatizing patients are inherently ambivalent. Their physical symptoms function as an ego-integrative principle and defense against intrapersonal disorganization. Accordingly, somatization helps maintain the appearance of ego integrity. This is an important point. Unlike the average patient whose daily functioning improves as their illness resolves, this is not generally the case with somatizers, particularly the chronic subtype. The alleviation of their symptoms is more often accompanied by psychological distress. They become more anxious, depressed, and eventually show signs of additional physical problems. Earlier we said that somatization is an illness that is indistinguishable from the patient. This becomes more evident when we look at the ways this population manages or, perhaps mismanages, ambivalence and progressive disorganizatioin. We will examine each of these concepts in turn.

AMBIVALENCE

The experience of having mixed feelings is a common one. So-called liminal periods, such as adolescence and midlife, in which persons undergo transitions from one life stage to another, are fraught with mixed feelings.[1] We often use the term "ambivalence" to identify our emotions at times like these, but psychologically speaking, ambivalence more accurately involves a sense of intrapsychic distress.[2] In relationships, ambivalence comes about when conflicting emotions are experienced toward the same person at the same time.[3] A patient feels torn between feelings of dependence and the developmentally appropriate desire to achieve independence and mature interpersonal functioning. Emotional conflict arises when separation from the other is perceived as an existential threat to survival. With adult patients, we often encounter situations in which separation from parents has either not occurred or has been avoided by dependence upon a parental substitute, such as a marital partner. The individual feels resentment, anger, or hostility toward the parental figure that s/he is unable to express because of fear of lost support and relational stability. S/he is betwixt and between: resentful of feeling dependent but, at the same time, unable to move toward mature adulthood without the support of the relationship. Where ambivalence remains outside conscious awareness, it serves as a psychological defense against the anxiety of separation. When ambivalence begins to break down and the intrapersonal conflict becomes more and more evident, patient distress becomes almost palpable.

For the individual who is able to integrate opposites and accept the ambiguity that is inherent in human relationships, ambivalence can be resolved without resorting to defensive strategies.[4] Where this either does not or cannot take place, less mature defenses such as denial and splitting are employed. The individual preserves the goodness of the "other" by splitting off and repressing the desire for independence, while using denial to prevent conflicting emotions from reaching conscious awareness.

In some cases, depletion and/or detachment are observed in patients' response to ambivalence.[5] Depletion is characterized as a "loss of libidinal energy."[6] "Libido" is a Freudian term which describes the energy that motivates and drives human activity. The signs of depleted libido are very similar to those we now call the neurovegetative symptoms of depression and include sleep and appetite disturbance, diminished sex drive, and anhedonia. With depletion, conflicted emotions that cannot be expressed openly within the context of a relationship are turned reflexively onto oneself. When these emotions are internalized, the eventual outcome is a situational depression; that is, depressive symptoms that have a specific and, as is often the case with ambivalence, an interpersonal etiology. It is not uncommon for these patients to seek antidepressant treatment in the mistaken belief that their symptoms have nothing to do with the relational issues. Predictably, however, even when antidepressant medication has restored emotional energy, unresolved and ambivalent feelings tend to remain intact. In an attempt to lessen the accompanying stress and anxiety, persons frequently turn to substance abuse or other maladaptive coping strategies.

Interestingly enough, antidepressant medication may sometimes complicate the clinical picture. When we fail to recognize the patient's symptoms as a defensive response to ambivalence and treat them solely as evidence of a mood disorder, we can actually reinforce the patient's defensive posture. Once the patient has obtained symptomatic relief, the unresolved ambivalence will eventually stimulate another depletive response and the depression will return. As a consequence, we not only have a patient who continues to suffer, we also have a secondary diagnosis which complicates treatment. Failure to address ambivalence results in a vicious circle that ultimately gets doctor and patient nowhere. Matching psychotropics with interpersonal psychotherapy is a more creative solution that poses a better treatment outcome.

Detachment is a distancing mechanism. By using denial, withdrawal, or avoidance, the individual reduces the anxiety that comes from feeling trapped in an ambivalent relationship.[7] Rather than admitting angry feelings, for example, an individual practices either distancing or numbing techniques to prevent anger from entering conscious awareness. We often see this behavior with patients who rush into new relationships to avoid dealing with uncomfortable mixed feelings about a spouse or lover. In essence, detachment allows individuals to ignore their feelings, while depletion internalizes them. In either case, the unresolved ambivalence is held in tension while the accompanying anxiety is reduced.

Whether one uses detachment or depletion seems to depend on temperament or personal predisposition. Individuals who seem shy and introverted, or have difficulty showing emotion, are probably more prone to depletion. Extraverted or more emotionally expressive personalities may be inclined to use detachment. We observe a dynamic between these two coping styles when the "detaching person" is inescapably confronted with their flight from reality and retreats into depletion and depressive symptomology. The "detaching personality" may actually fit the profile of the classic somatizer when s/he tries to deny the reality with which s/he is faced until denial becomes untenable and then s/he resorts to despair, depression, and physical symptomology as coping devices.

As noted above, ambivalence results from a desire to hold two conflicting feeling attitudes in tension: One needs the support of a dependency-type relationship while, at the same time, one wishes to achieve independent, adult functioning. In the mind of the individual, the latter cannot be achieved without completely losing the former. The young bird cannot fly without leaving the nest and, if it is to fly, it must leave the nest. Frustrated by indecision, the individual begins to resent his or her inability to leave and blames the supportive other for that failure. Further unable to address his or her negative feelings, s/he resorts to depletion or detachment to cope with the situation. Ambivalence protects against the tremendous fear and anxiety of losing the supportive relationship, as well as the fear that one will never "fly." In each case, ambivalence serves as a defense against emotional pain.

In his discussion of human motivation, Smith argues that "everything we do in life, no matter what it might be, is done in order to rid ourselves of a distressful feeling of some kind."[8] The difficulty with this position is we often prefer to assign noble motives to human behavior. The idea of a soldier throwing himself upon a grenade to save his comrades seems to us the highest form of heroism. One is reminded of the axiom, "Greater love hath no man than this, that a man lay down his life for his friends."[9] Nevertheless, Smith argues that behaviors such as this are intrinsically motivated by the desire to avoid the pain of guilt the soldier might experience should he leap to safety and allow his friends to perish. The point can be made that there is insufficient time to consider the fine points of psychology when the grenade is ticking toward explosion. Yet, stories of war are replete with examples of individuals who have experienced tremendous guilt for having survived when others died in battle. When the World Trade Center was attacked on September 11, 2001, two men who worked in one of the towers were among the thousands killed there. What makes those two men remarkable is that one of them could have escaped the building, but his wheelchair-bound coworker could not. The able-bodied man refused to leave the other behind and died with him rather than leave him. The able-bodied man surely did love his handicapped friend. In fact, he loved him so much that the thought of leaving him alone in that burning building was distressful enough that he would rather die than spend the rest of his life enduring the thought of having abandoned him.[10] Following Smith's reasoning, when an individual maintains a painfully ambivalent position with respect to a valued other, s/he does so in order to withdraw from the pain of decision and the even greater pain of loss. Consciously or unconsciously, we choose the type of pain we find most tolerable. Discomforting as somatization may become, for some individuals, it is preferable to the distress that accompanies the resolution of ambivalence, albeit, on an unconscious level. Chayes observes that persistently ambivalent positions can potentially result in a loss of part of the ego.[11] As we will point out later, diminished ego functioning is powerfully implicated in the development of somatization.

Depletion and detachment, as maladaptive coping styles for dealing with ambivalence, give us a clue as to how we can think about somatization as a defense against ambivalence. Insofar as somatization is an internalizing process, we can regard it as a depletive response to fears of abandonment and entrapment. The individual believes she cannot leave the nest because her wings fail to work properly. Accordingly, neither she nor the supportive relationship is responsible for her failure to achieve her dream of independence. On the contrary, the blame, if such exists, lies in her body and it falls to the clinician to resolve the ambivalence, if s/he dares. Furthermore, as long as the patient is disabled, such as by postoperative pain, she is freed from having to address her still-unresolved ambivalence. Once again, somatization transforms an interpersonal conflict into an intrapersonal one.

Unresolved dependency gives us some genuine insight into the processes underlying somatization, but our concern here is much broader than this single issue. In point of fact, we encounter somatizers in many different walks of life. The common element among them is the perception of an existential threat that stimulates the use of ambivalence as a defensive measure. Consider, for example, the exceedingly confident CEO who has prided himself on his success as a "self-made man." Mistakenly anticipating an immediate return to work postoperatively, he discovers to his chagrin, that he is unable to do so and finds himself more dependent on the assistance of others than he has ever been in his life. Dependency needs, common to all humans, have been a source of shame to our CEO and he has studiously avoided awareness of them at all costs; now, they are unavoidable. Torn between the necessity of depending on other persons and his desire to maintain independent functioning, he begins experiencing treatment-refractory postoperative pain. By transforming his ambivalence into symptoms of illness, the CEO—no doubt angrily—has found a way to transfer responsibility for his dependence to his body and preserve his self-image as a man who "needs no one." When asked how he feels about his reliance on others, he states he feels guilty but his behavior points to shame as the motive for somatization.

We understand shame and guilt to represent two differing emotional states. Guilt results from a sense of having violated a personal or social norm, of having committed an offense or trespass. Guilt is the violation of conscience and motivates confession, deserves punishment, and is relieved by acceptance and forgiveness. Guilt is about what we do. Shame, on the other hand, is about who we are and motivates concealment. While guilt demands restitution, shame hides behind somatization, and especially so when another individual's acceptance is doubtful. The impact of shame is even greater in situational somatization because here the threat to personal identity is more profound.

Situational somatization thus provides a way of defending against the twin threats of shame and ambivalence, leaving the self in tact. But what about patients who chronically somatize? Situational and chronic somatization syndromes present a phenotypical problem; that is, they have similar clinical presentations but different etiologies. Situational somatization is an ego-alien experience and is hardly the "defense of choice" in ordinary life circumstances. For the chronic somatizer, however, somatization is an ego-syntonic defense and functions as a "core" around which the self is organized. Opera tionally speaking, the extent of somatization is proportional to the intensity of interpersonal ambivalence. Or, put differently, somatization is, at least in part, a function of ambivalence. As the inability to tolerate interpersonal ambivalence may be regarded as a measure of ego strength, somatization, as a defense against ambivalence, is also a function of ego strength. As we will discuss later, ego strength is an essential distinction between the chronic and situational types of somatization.

Situational and chronic somatization may also be understood to represent neurotic and characterological life styles, respectively, and both types are subject to "ambivalence anxiety." By ambivalence anxiety we mean the intuition that the self will be irreparably disabled by a given life circumstance. This is the essence of the perception of existential threat: I will cease to be my functional self; at best, I'll be insane, at worst, I'll die. The fear that one will no longer function normally is reinforced by the greater fear of "progressive disorganization."[12] Somatization serves as a defense against progressive disorganization, which is experienced by the situational somatizer as a constant, albeit unconscious, threat, against which all available psychic energies and defenses must be brought to bear.[13] The response to pressure exerted by the unconscious constitutes the vertical dimension of ambivalence.

Earlier in this chapter we defined ambivalence in terms of conflicted emotions about something or someone who is external to the individual. When we talk about the vertical dimension of ambivalence, we are referring to multilevel ambivalence. In this case, conflict is not interpersonal but intrapersonal. In his groundbreaking work on the interpersonal theory of personality, Leary describes personality in terms of several levels, one of the most interior of which is largely, if not entirely, preconscious.[14] While we shall discuss this concept at some length in succeeding chapters, for now we wish to make the point that multilevel ambivalence describes the conflicted relationship that somatizers experience with respect to psychic material that lies outside the realm of conscious awareness. When this material erupts into consciousness, the result is some type of progressive disorganization; that is, psychotic regression.

PROGRESSIVE DISORGANIZATION

Progressive disorganization refers to a kind of decompensation in which the ego moves from normal to abnormal functioning. Under the pressure of overwhelming emotions, the ego adopts a defensive posture and regresses to an earlier, perhaps more primitive, coping style. Generally, the movement toward disorganization is halted by one's usual defensive strategies. Whatever factors motivate the regression, they are not so severe that the individual's preferred defenses cannot intervene and restore rational functioning. A recovering alcoholic, for example, might be confronted with her youngest child's illness. Normally, she would be tempted to regress and resume active drinking. However, her recovery process has nurtured more mature coping devices such as anticipation, which allows her to prepare for problems in advance. She anticipates the stresses accompanying her need to provide additional care for her child and arranges for nursing assistance rather than allowing herself to become exhausted and seek solace in alcohol.

What happens, however, when an individual's primary defenses are unable to come to the rescue? Marty suggests that this is precisely what happens when progressive disorganization breaks through fragile ego structures with symptoms that seem to come from all directions at once.[15] We can describe this process by way of analogy. A peaceful but relatively weak nation is bordered by an aggressive and warlike neighbor who is always threatening invasion. Once hostilities are engaged, the invading army systematically disables its opponent's primary defenses. As the defender withdraws in the face of overwhelming odds, abandoned territory falls under the control of the invader. Eventually, with its "back to the sea," the defender is forced to make a last stand which is, finally, a matter of life and death.

In response to an ever-present "threat of invasion" by progressive disorganization, chronic somatizers generally take refuge in somatic regression that is reminiscent of the child at the oral stage of development during the first year of life. Somatization enables a reenactment of the mother-child relationship into which the patient longs to escape. The role of the "good mother" is filled by the clinician, whose treatment is understood by the patient to demonstrate faithful, loving care. In short, the patient yearns to experience an infantile dependency relationship that promises to restore and maintain ego stability.

Somatization becomes the organizing principle of the personality and progressive disorganization the symbol for the existential pressures of life with which the chronic somatizer feels unable to cope. The chronic somatizer needs progressive disorganization to make somatization possible and thus enable the mother-child nurturing relationship with the physician. This fact alone helps explain why treatment of chronic somatizers is so difficult: The treatment itself reinforces the perception of a nurturing relationship that will sustain ego functioning. Accordingly, the chronic somatizer solves the dilemma of confronting ambivalence by transferring his dependence to his relationship with the physician, who is charged with the task of helping him cope with physical symptoms. When the patient perceives the clinician as having failed them in some way, this is tantamount to a failure in the nurturing relationship resulting in a depressed and angry patient. Ironically, treatment success also means the loss of the nurturing relationship, which the patient cannot tolerate either.

Unlike the chronic somatizer, the situational type regards the loss of functioning through illness as a threat of major proportions. These are persons who value their ability to hold down jobs and contribute to society. In fact, their personal identity may be strongly tied to a sense of capability in the working world. One even wonders if these individuals spend their lives compensating, or perhaps over-compensating, for a fear of vulnerability. In any case, they tend to verbalize their concerns in terms of loss of occupational functioning, disability, and becoming "dependent." When faced with an injury (surgery, illness, emotional trauma) that the individual perceives as a narcissistic wound—that is, one that strikes at the heart of his or her personal identity—s/he tends to undergo a progressive disorganization of functioning that can result in social withdrawal and isolation, despair, and suicidal ideation. The perception of a narcissistic wound is practically equivalent to an existential crisis.

Psychological testing by the senior author utilizing the Paindex Test® and the Somatic Displacement Analysis® Screen has revealed weaknesses in ego functioning in somatizing patients. The chronic somatizer tends to have a poorly organized defensive structure—in fact, somatization is essentially the only effective ego defense available to these individuals. The reason for this phenomenon might be found in Rodin's suggestion that somatization is related to a tendency to be more aware of physical than psychological experiences.[16] A child's ability to incorporate emotional states into psychological structures depends on the presence of a parental figure who can identify and verbalize emotions. Children depend on parents, not only to validate their emotions, but for the words to make sense of them. In order to learn how to distinguish emotional and physical states, children need parents who will respond to each in kind. In the absence of parental guidance, the child may learn to respond somatically to situations that might, more appropriately, require a psychological response. Consequently, when faced with emotionally distressing situations in adulthood, these individuals primarily experience physical discomfort. Some writers have suggested that mistaking somatic states for emotional ones may contribute to the development of alexithymia or the inability to verbalize emotions.[17] We typically encounter this type of pathology in the patient who seems unable to explain the nature or extent of his or her pain and, instead, repeats over and over, "I just hurt." In any case, problems with correctly identifying emotional states points to a disruption in ego development, which we regard as a key element in the pathology of the somatizing patient.

Situational somatizers possess a somewhat better organized ego which allows them to actually appear functionally normal until circumstances trigger progressive disorganization. Situational somatizers tend to look healthier than they are. When their inherently delicate ego structures are victimized by the intrusion of progressive disorganization, we observe the gradual loss of ego functioning. When the individual can no longer experience and resolve ambivalence at multiple levels, the result can be somatization.

Whereas the chronic somatizer uses somatization as a primary organizing principle of the personality, the situational somatizer uses it as an alternate organizing principle to be employed when all other defensive mechanisms have fallen in the path of progressive disorganization. In a final "retreat to the body," the individual—desperately and unconsciously—attempts to restore some sense of order to psychic chaos. Physical symptoms or somatic complaints become a lifeline which prevents the person from drowning in overwhelming anxiety and/or psychosis. Accordingly, we should resist the temptation to minimize somatization as a so-called neurotic response to stress. Patients present with situational somatization syndrome because they perceive, albeit unconsciously, that they have no other recourse to prevent total psychological breakdown. For the situational somatizer, it really has come down to a matter of life or death, where "death" is understood as the loss of self-esteem.

By now it should be clear that, although situational somatizers are always vulnerable to progressive disorganization, they do not experience it except under special circumstances. In the absence of an event which carries the weight of a narcissistic wound or existential threat, the ordinary defense mechanisms will hold fast and preserve normal functioning. The chronic somatizer, on the other hand, seems to undergo progressive disorganization as a factor in their normal experience. The persistent movement toward decompensation in the presence of life stressors results in the similar persistence of somatic complaints.

One of the most well-known descriptions of ambivalence is found in Shakespeare's *Hamlet: The Prince of Denmark*:

> To be, or not to be—that is the question:
> Whether 'tis nobler in the mind to suffer
> The slings and arrows of outrageous fortune
> Or to take arms against a sea of troubles,
> And by opposing end them. To die—to sleep
> No more; and by a sleep to say we end
> The heartache, and the thousand natural shocks
> That flesh is heir to . . .
> But that the dread of something after death—
> The undiscover'd country, from whose bourn
> No traveller returns—puzzles the will,
> And makes us rather bear those ills we have
> Than fly to others that we know not of?
> Thus conscience does make cowards of us all.[18]

Torn between his perceived duty to the ghost of his father and the fearfulness of the action he must undertake to punish his murderous uncle, Hamlet is in emotional torment. He has sworn that he will avenge his father's death but as the play progresses, Hamlet is hesitant to act. He is haunted by indecision and even death seems an unsatisfactory balm for his agony. Hamlet is Everyman and his struggle mirrors that of all persons who must recognize and reconcile painfully conflicted emotions. The Oxford don, C. S. Lewis, commented, "I would not cross the room to meet Hamlet. It would not be necessary. He is always where I am."[19]

Ambivalence and the underlying threat of progressive disorganization are critical elements for explaining why somatization can be quite treatment-resistant. Patients rock back and forth on an emotional teeter-totter, unable to decide which side to fall upon. Their desire to improve and their "reluctance or inability to confront . . . hidden feelings are often at complete loggerheads."[20] To change or not to change is the question; whether to remain in misery or leap into the unknown without a net. Either way, Hamlet lives again.

Chapter Five

Perception and Multilevel Perceptual Diagnosis

Somatization is an ego problem. In this regard, it is helpful to remember Freud's statement that the ego is, first of all, a "body-ego," which we understand to mean our primary sense of individuality is inextricable bound up with our awareness of ourselves as embodied persons. Thus we can speak of an embodied ego. Freud also emphasized that the conscious mind processes information from sensory (perception) to motor (activity), while in the unconscious dream state, this direction is reversed. Freud eventually dropped this topographic theory of the difference between the direction of thought between conscious and unconscious states. This development was quite likely due to the fact that his topographic theory had its origin in his *Interpretation of Dreams*, his foremost interest at the time, and the fact that there were few, if any, somatizers in his neurotic patient population. Yet this theory offers a precise explanation of the pre-psychotic state often seen in the chronic somatizer. In the pre-psychotic state, ego boundaries are often blurred with the result that the ongoing conscious state of sensory to motor can readily be reversed in the regressed state. This explains somatization as not only a defense against further regression but also as the amplification and prolongation of disturbingly painful and discomforting perceptions of one's basic sensory experience. Accordingly, we can say the pain associated with somatization is more perception than actual physical sensation. Perception and ego integration are not mutually exclusive; on a functional level they are mutually determined. This is not to say somatizing patients misinterpret bodily sensations but rather they mis-assign the meaning of physical distress and lack the ego-integration to correctly identify its source.

THE ROLE OF PERCEPTION

Our convictions regarding the validity of thinking about somatization in terms of perception have their origin in the senior author's (Smith) experiences while working at a state mental hospital a number of years ago.

> Before committing myself to years of graduate study, I wanted to get some real-life exposure to the field of clinical psychology. I must admit, I learned more from my experiences in this psychosocial microcosm working with patients, their physicians, nurses, and others, than at any other time in my professional educational experience. Keep in mind, this period in my life predates the advent of phenothiazines by seven years and predates, by even more years, the approval of lithium as a psychiatric treatment. I consider myself to have been most fortunate to have seen psychotic patients in their unvarnished state—an experience that students are now largely, if not entirely, denied. In this clinical setting, I interviewed and observed patients, administered multilevel tests and protocols, studied psychopathology in the texts of the time, and discussed my patients over and over with advanced interns and staff members. Over time, I became familiar with my patients' behavioral nuances and body language as well as their specious, tangential, and regressed thinking.
>
> In those days, the wards were very large and filled with up to forty or fifty psychotic patients at one time. Although the attending physicians were dedicated and sensitive individuals, they were generally too few in number to manage a ward on high ozone or lunar days. One wild, hallucinating patient shouting curses and counterinvectives at his interior "voices" was all that was needed to reduce the entire unit to bedlam. To short-circuit this escalation, the attendants would quietly and as unobtrusively as possible take the patient aside where he would be administered an intramuscular dose of sulfur and oil to the gluteal muscles. Almost at the moment of injection, the frenzied patient began to calm down and, subsequently, so did the rest of the ward.
>
> Fifty years ago, clinicians scarcely thought about somatization when there were so many psychotics, hysterics, disturbed neurotics, and manipulative psychopaths demanding attention. In those days, characterological disorders had yet to come in vogue. However, over the last few years, "sulfur and oil" has resurfaced in my thinking about somatization. In the case of our wildly psychotic patients, hallucinations were brought under control by means of an induced pain experience which halted the regression and served to provide the patient with an alternative, distracting focus about which to organize a weak ego. Admittedly, this distraction lasted only a few hours, but it certainly served its purpose.

The corollary we wish to draw with respect to somatization is if the decompensation of a weak ego can be controlled short-term, with focused, induced pain, it is just as easily imaginable how a pre-psychotic somatizer might shore up a vulnerable ego with a chronic somatic focus. Clearly, somatization is an unconscious process; that is a given. The vulnerable ego defends against the threat of decompensation by transferring psychological vulnerability onto somatic targets. Thus, somatization forms a protective cocoon against the possibility of a psychotic regression that threatens to release the patient's inner chaos. Over time, somatization becomes a way of life.

The somatizing patient's response to sensation is, of course, idiosyncratic; any response depends on the highly individualized awareness that something has occurred. Likewise, perception reflects a uniqueness that is often difficult to translate verbally. For example, we use such terms as stabbing, dull, aching, and so forth to describe the experience of pain, and we ask patients to rate their pain on a scale of 1 to 10, from complete absence to excruciating pain. Helpful as this approach may be, it still falls short of communicating the perception of pain with absolute clarity. Even if persons felt pain identically, their perceptions of it would differ because perception is the outcome of cerebral processing, rather than sensory inputs.

Using functional imaging, Singer et al. have shown that empathy for persons in distress activates only that portion of the pain network associated with affective qualities, not sensory ones.[1] In their study, bilateral anterior insula, rostral anterior cignulate cortex, brainstem, and cerebellum were activated, not only when subjects received a painful sensation, but also by a signal that alerted them to the fact that a loved one experienced pain.[2] Activity in the anterior insula and anterior cingulate cortex correlated with empathy, while activity in the posterior insula/secondary somatosensory cortex, the sensorimotor cortex, and the caudal anterior cignulate cortex were specific to the experience of receiving pain.[3] To put this more simply, one's ability to imagine how a painful sensation might feel is the basis for understanding and relating to another's potential response to pain. This may seem elementary, but here we have evidence based on neuroimaging that sensation is highly individualized; we really don't know how another person feels, but we imagine how we might feel in similar circumstances. In short, sensation is generalizable on an imaginal level, not an experiential one.

Perception is no less subject to individual considerations because it depends on interpretation and interpretation reflects experiences that tend to be unique to the individual.[4] Thus, perception is not only a creative act by which we transform sensory inputs into meaningful information, it is also the means by which we transform the reality of any experienced object.[5] Accordingly, perception involves attention. The interpersonal theorist, Harry Stack Sullivan, described selective inattention as the patient's tendency to avoid subjects that were perceived as inherently anxiety provoking.[6] Thus, perception is not only an attentional process, but also a discriminating one. One of the main features of Donald Nathanson's affect theory is its emphasis upon affect as a primary, neurobiological experience.[7] Affect tells us that something has entered our awareness and is vying for our attention. Emotion is generated as the outcome of selective attention paid to affect as representative of experience. Perception is the process of selectively attending to sensory stimuli that the individual finds inherently meaningful. Consequently, one might say that "while perception screens our sensations, memory screens our perceptions (and thus) only those perceptions are selected and integrated into one's world picture have any value for him in (terms of) emotional response."[8] Perception, then, is the critical element in the evaluation of experience because it provides the criterion by which we subjectively arrange the elements of our experience in a way that makes sense to us.

Our vocabulary for conceptualizing perception has grown from sensation to include selective attention, interpretation, and the assignment of meaning on both conscious and unconscious, symbolic levels. In the language of traditional psychology, the perception of reality was primarily a matter of sensory awareness. Reality is concrete and encountered through the medium of the five senses. Anything that is not sensibly apprehended is either nonexistent or simply imaginary. Perception of reality is the "awareness of things that exist, in opposition to imagination, which is a creation of things that do not exist."[9] Reality could thus be defined as matter; that is, that which has mass and takes up space. More recently, we have come to understand that reality cannot be so narrowly limited. Much of our understanding of cosmology, for example, depends on theoretical constructs that interpret physical reality in more fluid terms. Depth psychology has taught us to attend to psychic materials whose effects are exerted outside of conscious awareness. In other words, reality does not have to be limited solely to the realm of conscious experience.

It is the relationship between the constitutive elements of a thing combined with the conscious and unconscious perceptions of the observer that really defines existence.[10] Of course, when we talk about conscious and unconscious perceptions, we're referring to the interpretive and meaning-making process in which individuals engage when perception takes place. As Werner Wolff reminds us, appearance and existence are not necessarily identical concepts. Appearance can mask existence: The apparently satisfied and content individual may, in fact, be profoundly dissatisfied and unfulfilled.[11] Accordingly, existence is dependent upon interpretation and interpretation is very much intertwined with unconscious projection. Wolff observes,

> Not every perception becomes a subjective symbol for us; only those objects upon which we project images or ideas do. Potentially, every object can become an existential perception. . . . Most of these projections have no deep effect upon our psychological organization. Some projections, however, may change

> our entire outlook on life. They challenge our existence. . . . These challenging perceptions we call existential perceptions.[12]

Perception and interpretation are inseparable aspects of the assignment of meaning to experience. Yet, we aren't talking about an entirely conscious process because meaning-making is often the result of unconscious projections.

In projection, unpleasant or unacceptable intrapsychic contents are unconsciously attributed to others. One is thereby permitted to disown those aspects of oneself and "hate" them in someone else. Projection is a powerful element in human experience and it occurs in collective, as well as, individual instances. For example, former president Ronald Reagan labeled the Soviet Union as an "evil empire," thus permitting a collective split between good and evil. Instead of recognizing how all persons and/or nations are capable of blameworthy behavior, such a split enables one collective body to disavow itself of prejudice, greed, and other negative labels. By so doing, Americans could identify themselves with patriotic and humanitarian values and the Soviet Union with opposition to those values. Projection, however, is not merely a defense mechanism. We unconsciously project our own humanity onto other individuals, for example, enabling us to relate to them as distinct persons. Thus, while all projections are significant for the organization of personality, some have profound effects and may result in deep psychic disturbance.

Just as the resolution of ambivalence requires us to reconcile opposing emotions, appearance and interpretation must be united in order to perceive reality as it is. The inability to do so is reflected in somatization. When we respond to another person with a sense of inexplicable revulsion, interpretation is split off from appearance; our feelings are grounded in unconscious projection rather than a real-life perception. Wolff notes, "By splitting the appearance and the interpretation . . . the mind tries to free itself from the impact that a certain happening has upon it. Depriving the happening of its meaning or interpretation means that it cannot play a role in the conscious organization of personality. However, the meaning is split only from consciousness—it perseveres in the unconscious."[13] We either repress the event or the meaning assigned to it; in either case, the repressed material tends to become dominant in the psychological makeup of the person.

In somatization, the dominant unconscious element becomes an unconscious pattern of somatic displacement. The repressed interpretation of a single experience can "produce a new unconscious interpretation of all (experiences) and create an unconscious picture of the world which is different from our conscious one."[14] Somatization thus represents an idea of life experience that stands outside conscious awareness. The patient presents with a conscious awareness of diffuse pain and malaise which reflects disturbances in perception that can be traced to similar disturbances in the perception of his or her psychological experience. Certain inward expectations may actually provoke changes in the body ego. Accordingly, somatization is the outcome of inner psychological disturbance that is somatically displaced and experienced as physical symptomology. While we typically think of this taking place in the situational somatizer, the fact is that chronic somatizers are no less vulnerable to the need and/or desire to find symptomatic relief from the psychological pain of a poorly developed ego by turning to the body for release.

If we think back to the observations described earlier in this chapter, we can now understand the function of sulfur in oil and the psychological focus provided by physical pain. For those patients, the experience of psychosis was tremendously distressing. The shift of attention from taunting inner voices, suspicion, and fear was a welcome respite, and in retrospect, we can say the body came to their rescue and restored ego functioning, if only for a short time. Although the pre-psychotic personality structure in chronic somatizers is not as readily apparent as may be observed in schizophrenic or bipolar patients, the shift of focus to the body has the same effect as sulfur in oil. Metaphorically speaking, we might even say that somatization is sulfur in oil, particularly in view of what it accomplishes. Somatic symptoms rescue the individual from the threat of psychotic disintegration and provide an anchor in something conceived as tangible, dependable, and real. The nature of somatization renders this process outside conscious awareness, but the tenacity with which somatizing patients cling to their symptoms is clear evidence that, for them, their individuality, their personhood, is at stake.

Thus, it is in mental processing that we find the key to understanding how patients can experience delays in surgical recovery or chronic pain and avoid falling into the trap of suggesting that these problems are imaginary. It is one thing to talk about emotional stresses finding expression in physical illness and quite another to talk about the intentional role played by the mind in the development of physical symptoms, and in the case of somatization, this is precisely what we are suggesting. The mind, as that neurobiological amalgam that interacts to form the decision-making, information-processing, reflective, feeling, and relating entity that is a human personality, exerts a symptom-generating influence on the body and drives individual behavior.

How may we apply this line of thinking to patients who appear to have abnormalities in neural processing? For example, Glass has studied self-reported cognitive problems in patients with fibromyalgia. She notes that nearly all patients with fibromyalgia have "central processing abnormalities; central augmentation of sensory input may interfere with other activities involved in processing sensory input and the ability to ignore items that are distracting and maintain focus on what is important."[15] In these patients perception may be skewed by central nervous system augmentation of sensory inputs resulting in selective attention focused on painful sensations. Chronic pain induces an affective response associated with anxiety which increases the patient's attentional focus on distressing physical sensations and reducing their ability to concentrate on alternate subject matter. Abnormalities in central processing may in fact predispose these patients to experience distortions in perception resulting in a self-definition that centers on painful sensations. Instead of regarding the patient's perceptions as evidence of cognitive distortion, creative treatment strategies might better focus on re-education of the mechanism of perception, enabling patients to redefine their experience.

MULTILEVEL PERCEPTUAL DIAGNOSIS

The predominant and discouraging element noted in many studies concerning somatization results from a focus on descriptive phenomena that disregards the internal dynamics of personality disorganization and multiple levels of variability. The introduction of sensory perceptual distortion from an existential viewpoint provides us with not only the necessary terminology, but also a context within which to approach a meaningful dynamic study of the somatization process, that is, a much needed systematic and operationally defined framework designed to separate intrapsychic variability indices of behavior. A useable tool which relates levels of expressed behavior with exigencies of clinical decision making would be a valuable aid for the practitioner.

Our approach to intrapersonal factors is based on the personality theory devised by Leary more than fifty years ago. His original concept was designed to predict change occurring in the course of interpersonal psychotherapy. We have applied these diagnostic and prognostic features in the framework of an intrapsychic system to be used in a medical somatization clinic and treatment center with medical and surgical patients. One of the core tests we use to determine a diagnosis of somatization is the Paindex® test, which predicts probabilities for successful outcome of treatment aimed at pain relief. Our practice is to administer the Paindex® test, and once the presence and extent of somatization has been determined, the SDA Screen® (Somatic Displacement Analysis) is administered to elucidate multilevel variability in intrapersonal conflict for treatment planning. This additional data enables us to decide whether we are dealing with chronic or situational somatization.

For persons unfamiliar with Leary's multilevel scheme, we would like to refer to it briefly—a more extended discussion will follow in the next chapter. According to Leary, personality is divided into five conceptual levels, each expressing different aspects of an individual's presentation and manner of functioning in the world. Level I refers to public perception and includes the clinician's impressions of the patient which are derived from the intake interview as well as the patient's public communication or symptom expressions. Level II relates patients' conscious self-report of themselves as persons. Level III concerns private perceptions; that is, preconscious imagery. Level IV represents the total repression as detected by the significantly omitted aspects of personality noted by the patient's inattention or avoidance. Finally, level V represents the personal values, the ego ideal, the type of person the patient would most like to be.[16]

The clinical interview largely reveals Level I information about symptom complaints insofar as they are observed by the clinician. Factors such as body language, facial expression, vocal tone, and word selection are important factors in creating a clinical impression. Level I, of course, presents the public and social impact patients have on other individuals, and in this case, the interviewing clinician. In a sense, Level I represents the clinician's experience of the patient and the presenting complaints. Comments derived from family members also represent types of Level I interaction and contribute to the clinician's understanding of the patient, but primarily at this level. Level II presents more than the patient's self-report; it is really a description of the patient's perception of his/her own experience.

The extent of pain or disability, social and occupational dysfunction, the history of failed attempts at treatment—all these are described in terms which are intended to suggest the most accurate rendering of the patient's experience. Clinical interviews which cease with Level I and II material characterize the most common form of initial doctor-patient interaction. In typical parlance, we might refer to Level I as signs and Level II as symptoms. However, if we wish to gain a more accurate picture of the patient, we compare Level II material with Level III, the patient's preconscious imagery, which enables direct comparison between two levels providing evidence of multilevel variability of conflicts. Level III is assessed through different levels of projective test data which taps into fantasy material which lies just outside the patient's conscious awareness. Level IV is even more elusive since it involves in unexpressed unconscious which is repressed and is totally outside conscious awareness; that is, Level IV material is determined by the patient's selective inattention and total avoidance. Although not specifically diagnostic, Level IV information may be useful later on in psychological therapy.

The usefulness of level V material (ego ideal) in understanding somatization becomes clear when the patient insists that, since their self-description (II) and level V are the same, completing level V is useless repetition. Essentially, the patient is saying their self-experience and their imagined ideal life are identical.

Rejection of the notion that there might be a variance between life as the patient experiences it and life as they might wish to experience it tells use a great deal about the patient's enormous rigidity, inflexibility, and inability to tolerate any sort of change which might result from psychological treatment.

In addition to rigidity and resistance to change, the potential for progressive disorganization and regression has a direct effect on the decision-making process of the clinician. Multilevel perceptual analysis offers much more promise than reliance upon Level I and Level II material alone for prediction in our dynamic investigation. Rather than concentrating on one level at a time in isolation, we have a system of dynamic interplay. One should be reminded that personal perceptions of the patient are restricted to Level I and thus, one's data is only partially reflective of the patients level of insight and cooperation as an historian. To complete Level II only, an objective test such as Paindex® will establish the clear presence and level of intensity of somatization.

Paindex® and the SDA Screen® are designed and employed as operationally defined procedures assuring that all behavior levels are consistent with evidence-based medicine. Once behavioral levels are determined, the system is set, or locked. The structural stability is defined and its flexibility determined and predicted for future behavior.

We mentioned the comparison of Level II with Level III provides evidence of the multilevel variability of conflicts. The variability dimension is a category for classification. It taps similarity, dissimilarity, flexibility for change, conflict, and discrepancy at the various levels, such as through repression, suppression, displacement, projection of one's own behavior and ambivalence versus consistency, whether defensive or adaptable, successful or unsuccessful, rigid or inflexible, and so forth. Variability indices offer an entirely new departure in multilevel diagnosis as it deals with conflicts, inconsistencies, and discrepancies which are the essence of dynamic psychology but at the same time offer complex barriers to development of personality theory in general and the understanding of somatization in particular. The multilevel diagnostic phenomena reflects the dynamics of organization as well as progressive disorganization, whether the latter is transient or a fixed pathological state. These dynamics appear in constellations of recognizably distinct somatizing syndromes, whether chronic or situational, as well as varied patterns of non-somatizing conflicted patients, including malingered somatization records.

The multilevel diagnostic system reflects hierarchical patterns at different levels of behavior which provide answers to functional diagnostic questions about the patient's motivation and subsequent treatment. For example, during the intake interview what they patient says or does, or indirectly expresses, tells us something about the patient's rigidity of security operations, their type and degree of severity, and their ambivalence or conflicts. Adding information from Level II to the clinician's Level I impressions has an exponential effect. For example, the patient may give a fearful passive dependent impression during symptomatic impression at Level I but the self-report presents the patient as confident and independent, a combination which is now packed with meaning. Here the double diagnostic analysis is useful in pointing up the discrepancy or conflict in the patient's presenting façade, indicating marked misrepresentation by the patient of the effect of his symptom or ambivalence in the patient's motivation.

When we add Level III to any diagnostic formula we gain even more empirical information which assists us in making predictions about future behavior because it gives us a more meaningful pattern. Actually, the third level of behavior is of particular clinical interest since it helps explain the shifts that occur between levels I and II, that is, surface behavior of overt presentation and conscious self-description as predictive of future behavior. For example, a patient who expresses overly conventional and friendly behavior at levels I and II may indicate a shift in the preconscious Level III of considerable concern with hostility. This is a pattern often seen with somatizers, that is, an underlying pattern of antisocial feelings exists beneath the façade of bland overly conventional presentation. Level IV involves themes attributed to the fantasy of others, a level not clinically studied due to its lack of specific significance, yet on occasion, it gives some hints as to how rigid or flexible the entire personality pattern is and what behavior may be tolerated in others but is ignored in the self. This factor is helpful in predicting patient behavior in treatment involving dialectics or group therapy sessions.

The question of malingering, of course, must be addressed, in spite of several validity scores in the Paindex® scale to assist in its detection. Findings suggestive of malingering are an interesting phenomenon. The senior author has seen many patients on referral by internists, gastroenterologists, and so forth to evaluate the patient's proclivity for somatization in view of ongoing complaints of pain in the absence of positive clinical and laboratory findings. In the event no evidence of somatization was forthcoming from the test administration, the decision that other motivating influences might be implicated was generally left to the discretion of the referring physician in consultation with the patient. In most cases, referral for Paindex® evaluation expressed the physician's desire to rule out somatization when all other potential diagnostic possibilities had been exhausted. Once the diagnosis of last resort had been eliminated, other clinical decisions would be indicated. However, it is the senior author's opinion that test profiles that result from testing attitudes expressed by "I can't or I won't" responses, or profiles distorted by legitimate personality pathology or malingering, may be suggested but not conclusively determined by any test. Instead, the final determination must result from an evaluation of incongruities in the patient's functioning, and that, of course, falls under the aegis of the attending physician.

The multilevel analysis diagnostic system provides for a great number and variety of behavior types, which leads to more refined clinical decisions. The process whereby diagnosis is determined can also be utilized in decision making for follow-up treatment. The latter, measured by the same theoretical framework, offers the necessary evidence by which any aspects of this system can be evaluated in outcome studies.

The diagnosis of medically unexplained symptoms of somatization tends to be heavily influenced by the patient's multilevel perceptual variability organization. The specific type of organization provides the diagnostician with critical information reflecting the quality of ego-integrity or the lack thereof, which is a central issue involved in understanding the mind-body interface. In the following chapter, we will discuss the personality organizations we believe are more frequently encountered in somatization. The constellation of behavioral dynamics within perceptual levels provides us with vital information about the patient's idiosyncratic translation of expectations into realities. We now turn to the practical application of the multilevel system of diagnosis in the process of relating to the somatizing patient.

Chapter Six

Dealing with Impasse Resistance

In previous chapters we have discussed how relationships with the somatizing patient can be impaired by factors such as clinician ambivalence and poor ego integrity. Other factors also come into play as doctor and patient attempt to interact in meaningful ways, including personality traits and communication style. Published research concerning personality and somatization is sparse, but in a fairly recent study, Hakula et al. found that somatizing patients tend to show signs of low novelty-seeking and high harm-avoidance behaviors.[1] Somatizing patients have been observed to communicate more psychological distress, functional impairment, and social isolation than non-somatizers.[2] Somatizers may also show indications of externally oriented or concrete thinking styles which are associated with alexithymia.

Alexithymia is a technical term that refers to difficulty identifying, verbalizing, and communicating emotional states. The extent to which alexithymia figures in somatization is a subject of mixed opinion. Kooiman et al. found that alexithymia did not play a significant role in their study of patients with unexplained medical symptoms.[3] Porcelli et al., on the other hand, observe that alexithymia is a reliable and stable predictor of treatment outcome in patients with functional gastrointestinal disorders. They suggest that clinicians might improve treatment outcomes by identifying patients with high alexithymia, and focusing on improving patient skills for coping with emotionally stressful situations.[4] Taylor et al. note that, compared to nonalexithymic patients, alexithymic ones demonstrate a fairly wide range of somatic symptoms and bodily concerns. In addition, they note that alexithymic patients possess less ego strength, more dependency, and are more likely to engage in impulsive and acting out behaviors.[5] Blaustein and Tuber point out that somatization may be "specifically and temporally linked with (an) inability to fully tolerate either (one's) longings for empathic connection to others, or the disappointments when those desires are not satisfied . . . (thus) the affective trigger for a psychosomatic eruption may have an intrinsic relational dimension."[6] The proclivity of somatizing patients to verbalize their distress in somatic terms may thus reflect an overall inability to verbalize feeling states in more abstract terms.

The problems the authors of this volume have observed in clinical practice point to personality factors and associated communication styles as critical elements in the treatment of somatization. This is especially the case when impasse resistance develops between patient and clinician. Resistance refers to aspects of patients' functioning that are intended to preserve the status quo in their psychological lives.[7] In light of our discussion of progressive disorganization, a patient's attachment to illness symptoms and inability to improve despite adequate treatment represents resistance. Impasse resistance is more serious and describes a situation in which the relationship between patient and clinician are at loggerheads. Everything the clinician has attempted has failed to penetrate the patient's resistance and now the relationship has become oppositional. To a great extent, we believe this state of affairs arises because the clinician is unaware of basic principles of personality theory as they can be applied to the somatizing population. In some cases, impasse resistance may be impossible to resolve without either the clinician making a referral or the patient dropping out of treatment. In many more cases, however, impasse resistance can be avoided. The first step in this direction involves learning how personality type predisposes some individuals to somatization.

PERSONALITY THEORY AND SOMATIZATION

Leary's penetrating insights into levels of personality functioning in the ambivalence and conflicts of the pre-psychotic patient are extremely applicable to our efforts to establish a working relationship with somatizing patients. Leary defined the common elements between psychosomatic and psychotic personalities through the use of a multilevel theory of identifying personality differences and demonstrated their pertinence in the evaluation of outpatients for psychotherapy.[8] Let's summarize what we've said previously about the multilevel system of personality diagnosis. First, Leary identifies five levels of personality. Level I relates to an individual's overt behavior as it is perceived by others; that is, the patient's impact on the clinician. Level II is comprised of an individual's self-report and gives us a picture of their self-perception. Level III is derived from preconscious, fantasy materials—dreams, projective tests, and the like—that suggest how individuals imagine themselves. These expressions of the self are called "preconscious" because they symbolize aspects of the personality which are not directly or consciously perceived by the individual. Level IV contains those aspects of the personality that are compulsively and inflexibly avoided by the individual. Level IV informs us about the rigidity of an individual's defensive system. Level V refers to the values one holds; that is, the interpersonal traits which one regards as good, proper, or morally correct. These diagnostic levels form a series of concentric circles, proceeding inward from Levels I through V. The name given each type reflects the overall manner in which the types adjust to interpersonal relationships and cope with anxiety.

Personality doesn't function on one level to the exclusion of the others. We are frequently more than we seem and societal perceptions may be at variance with our self-perceptions. An individual is described by his peers as brave and fearless while he sees himself as shy and withdrawing. These differences show that there is an interplay between the five levels that reveals personality organization. Leary describes this interplay in terms of the indices of variability, which refers to the "stability or variation existing among the levels of personality at one point in time."[9] Simply put, variability is built into the system: All personality levels vary with respect to one another. Some persons express more variability in personality than others, which is what we mean when we say that some individuals are more flexible and others possess a more rigid personality structure. Some are more amenable to change and adaptation and others are more resistant. Personality structure has both adaptive and defensive functions.

Not only do we observe structural variability between the levels of personality, we also observe temporal variability, which means that behavior changes over the life span.[10] Time invariably brings about changes in personality. Furthermore, there is situational variability that refers to differences in culture and environment.[11] Factors such as gender, age, national origin, social status, and so forth, figure in at this point. The decisive, hard-driving CEO may be the submissive spouse at home. Situational variability reflects more of our day-to-day experience as individuals in society.

Leary's indices of variability are very important to an understanding of somatization because they reveal a great deal about the nature of the somatizing ego, in particular its proclivity toward poor organization. When we talk about a weak ego, we're really talking about the structural stability of the personality. The somatizer frequently appears quite stable at Level I, but there is an underlying instability in the ego structure which undermines his or her ability to manage change and anxiety. In other words, there are interlevel discrepancies in the personality that can be predictive of the direction and amount of change that can be expected in the individual over time.[12] Broad inconsistencies, such as between the observations of others and our own self-report, are evidence of ego instability.

When there is considerable discrepancy between the clinician's observations (Level I), the patient's self-report (Level II), and their preconscious imagery (Level III), it is frequently due to an unconscious sense of shame about the Level III traits. Persons who find Level III traits unacceptable either take great pains to disavow them or to pejoratively ascribe them to others (projection). For example, individuals who pride themselves in their independence may express dependency in their preconscious imagery. Their unconscious shame is expressed in the manner in which they hold homeless persons up to derision. While a more conscious awareness and acceptance of one's dependency needs could balance the personality and lead to compassion and empathy, denial or repression of Level III traits only serves to reinforce one's rigidity. When this occurs, the discrepancy between the levels of personality contributes dramatically to ego instability. With this background in mind, we can use Leary's system to identify the four personality types that seem most prone to somatization: the overlyconventional, the hypernormal, the dependent, and the managerial-autocratic.

THE OVERLYCONVENTIONAL TYPE

The overlyconventional personality is marked by extroverted friendliness (Level I). Persons who demonstrate this character style "seem to be comfortable when they are evoking 'good feelings' and establishing harmonious, amicable relations with others."[13] Overlyconventionals are cooperative, agreeable, and seem more comfortable with socially accepted values. We enjoy overlyconventionals because they are cheerful, friendly, and make for pleasant company. These individuals like to describe themselves as "nice people" and they prefer the company of like-minded, "nice people."

Overlyconventionals dislike unpleasant or "angry" persons and often vehemently deny being angry themselves. Because they tend to deny their own needs in deference to those of others, they typically complain that no one notices their efforts or makes similar sacrifices on their behalf. Their disappointment and feelings of being neglected are often the source of a great deal of anger and resentment at Level III. They describe themselves as sad but their affect (Level I) says otherwise: they may raise their voices, use profanity, and appear angry. Overlyconventional fantasies include imagining themselves as direct, forceful, and unconcerned about the opinions of others. Nevertheless, once these fantasies are admitted, they are accompanied by denial: "Oh, but I would never actually do that!" The flip side of the overlyconventional is a rigid over-optimism that idealizes relationships and makes excuses for the behavior of other persons, even if this misrepresents the nature of an encounter. As a consequence, their range of interpersonal responses is rather narrow and they seem fearful of expressing themselves, especially if this means going against the values or opinions of their social group.

Pre-psychotic patterns of underlying sadism or mistrust are frequently observed in somatizing patients characterized by multilevel patterns of overconventionality. Leary observes:

> Whenever a patient presents a multi-level pattern which involves claimed conventional friendliness (Levels one and two) contrasted with a distrustful or a masochistic Level III score, the danger flag should be flown. This is a paranoid phenomenon. This pattern indicates poor motivation for therapy. The patient claims to be a normal persona and probably does not want his personality investigated or changed.[14]

The character pattern of overconventionality which serves so well interpersonally becomes a genuine liability in treatment. The fatal damage to the hull of the *Titanic* was located beneath the water line. So it is with multilevel personality patterns: The social persona seems functional enough, but the preconscious Level reveals the implicit danger. Twin studies have indicated that somatizers are often paired with an antisocial, nonsomatizing sibling.[15] Beneath the friendly exterior of the overlyconventional, we find the negative elements of the nonsomatizing twin which tend to be activated when the social façade is threatened. Psychotherapy presents a threat not only to one's perceived normality, but also to the character structure which defends against anxiety. Overlyconventional types with whom we have worked have difficulty understanding how it is possible they should require therapy when they invest so much effort in being socially acceptable. For example, a patient's question, "What's wrong with being nice?" reveals their reliance on an overlyconventional façade as a defense against therapeutic probing.

Somatization allows the overlyconventional to keep Level III hostility safely locked away from conscious awareness. Drawing upon evolutionary principles, Price et al. associate social submissiveness with the adoption of a sickness metaphor.[16] Instead of expressing dissatisfaction and conflict at a verbal level, some individuals use sickness to communicate submissiveness, since sickness implies weakness and elicits compassion from others.[17] The message they send is, "I'm too ill to stand up to you."

Thus, the sickness may take the form of "soldier's heart," or irritable bowel, or hyperventilation, or fits or faints or tremblings, or of a general prostration. From the point of view of decisions made at multiple levels, these do not represent forms of conscious deception or malingering (in which the sickness metaphor is used at the highest or rational brain level) because the individual truly believes that sickness exists; in fact, he or she is so convinced that any suggestion to the contrary receives violent rejection. This reaction has been observed when patients with chronic fatigue learn that the doctor considers them perhaps psychologically rather than physically ill. The metaphor of sickness depends on an archetypal recognition of the sick role, and since it likely evolved before recognition of depression as a legitimate reason for taking the sick role the metaphor therefore fails to include psychiatric disability. When a physician tells patients that they are not physically ill, they feel invalidated and not surprisingly reject the opinion.[18]

In fact, the patient may indeed be quite ill, but of course, his or her symptoms derive from psychological, rather than physical, disease processes. Somatization enables the overlyconventional to tell the clinician, in effect, "Not only am I too ill to confront others, I'm too ill to face myself."

We have stressed previously that somatizers are highly conventional people whose heightened ambivalence often underlies an overlyconventional façade. Chronic somatizers are quite accurately perceived as "difficult patients" when they are unwilling and/or unable to become involved in the kind of effective doctor-patient relationship that is necessary to "work through" the personality problems that predispose to somatization in the first place.

THE HYPERNORMAL TYPE

The hypernormal personality presents at Level I as "reasonable, successful, sympathetic, mature."[19] These individuals strive to avoid seeming weak or unconventional and, instead, stress their strength, self-confidence, and independence. These traits are most obvious in social situations where the hypernormal seeks to be helpful, supportive, and responsible with respect to other persons. When a neighbor is in trouble or has experienced a family crisis, hypernormals are quick to answer the call of duty and provide whatever assistance they can. They also place a high value on law and social structure (Level II). For example, when asked why she adhered to the speed limit in a school zone, one hypernormal answered, "Why, because there was a speed limit sign in clear view!" Unlike other types which might offer the presence of the police and the potential for punishment as motivations for restricting their speed, the hypernormal only requires an awareness of what is considered socially acceptable behavior. Their strong sense of duty and willingness to follow a chain of command renders hypernormality a desirable quality for military personnel.

Maladaptively, at Level III, the hypernormal is threatened by the prospect of appearing defeated, passive, dependent, unfriendly, or abnormal. Paradoxically, while these individuals will be quick to donate to charity out of a sense of social responsibility, they may also view socially disadvantaged individuals as lacking the drive or commitment to better themselves. In this way, their own Level III passivity and dependence is disavowed and projected outwardly. In the consultation room, the hypernormal tends to minimize symptoms; in point of fact, it is typically very difficult for hypernormal types to seek any kind of psychological treatment because of the implication that there is something "abnormal" about their behavior that requires professional attention.

With the hypernormal, it is helpful to remember their firmly entrenched defenses against "abnormality." Therapeutic interventions that suggest there might be a dysfunctional element at work in their values or approach to life are met with staunch denial. Like the overlyconventional, at Level III the hypernormal has a great deal of unconscious paranoia. When their strong, independent façade begins to break down, the first thing one sees is suspiciousness and distrust. As these repressed feelings generate increasing anxiety, the patient, sensing limited options, either resorts to depression, a "flight into health," or a search for long-term obsessive solutions to cope with their anxiety. With flight into health, the patient announces that the therapy has "worked," they are feeling better, and there is no longer any need for treatment. In essence, the patient "flees" the signs of illness and takes refuge in a façade of "health." Patients know intuitively that they can't return to a pre-therapy position; they become indecisive and panic sets in: They have to get out, there is too much anxiety. This is the point where somatization may become evident. As patients' hypernormal defenses give way one by one or perhaps all at once, they turn to somatization as the defense of last resort. With an inward sigh of relief, hypernormals reassure themselves that their problem is physical and the therapist obviously had no idea what was going on in the first place.

Consider the following clinical vignette. The CEO of a successful company went on a business trip to finalize an important deal. Anxious about flying, he took an antianxiety agent prescribed by his primary care physician. He reported that, at the time, he thought he was still feeling the effects of the medication when he went out to dinner with friends later that evening to celebrate his success. An occasional drinker, he had a couple of glasses of wine and reported feeling slightly intoxicated when it was suggested they attend a gentlemen's club for additional entertainment. While at the club, the patient had several more drinks and ended up having a liaison with one of the dancers. Upon returning home, he found himself feeling terribly guilty and fearful that he might have contracted a sexually transmitted disease. Despite negative results from a thorough battery of tests, he was convinced that he must have an infection, and he obtained consults from other physicians over a period of several weeks. One of these suggested a hepatitis injection, and the patient agreed.

Unable to accept any reassurance that he was quite well, the patient became depressed and increasingly anxious and was referred for a psychiatric evaluation. In the course of the interview, the patient reiterated his primary problem was ongoing pain at the injection site. He had studied his "condition" on the Internet and was convinced that his depression must be related to his unresolved pain. He reported that he had "forgiven himself" for his lapse of marital infidelity and believed his wife had done likewise. Nonetheless, he was unable to sleep and he obsessed about his condition to the point that he was unable to work or function normally at home. Ordinarily a highly responsible and respected individual in his personal and professional relationships, he was baffled by what had taken place on the business trip and could only attribute his behavior to peer pressure. While discussing his physical symptoms, he frequently looked around suspiciously and he admitted he suspected other people were talking about him behind his back. An atypical antipsychotic medication was prescribed and he began psychotherapy. Therapy revealed the patient's long-standing belief that his worth as a person was closely tied to his ability to perform responsibly in life. At the same time, he gradually admitted he had fantasized about doing something forbidden, something he believed other men who lacked his moral convictions were free to do. His normal inhibitions diminished by a combination of alcohol and the medication, the patient's Level III rebelliousness surfaced and he got himself in trouble.

Interestingly, while he could admit the nature of his behavior on the trip, he was unable to connect his physical pain with his resistance to examining his sense of guilt and shame. When therapy threatened to address these issues, he retreated to the pain in his arm and insisted he would be less depressed if he was only no longer in pain. Progress was finally made when therapy began to focus on the patient's fear that his pain was evidence of a lethal illness. For this obsessive hypernormal, yielding to his unconscious desire to rebel carried with it the threat of personal dissolution or ego death. By examining the existential fear of death, the patient was enabled to eventually confront his guilt and obtain relief from his physical discomfort. Clearly, this vignette describes a case of situational somatization triggered by ambivalence with respect to Level III ambitions and concurrent shame and guilt about having yielded to their influence.

THE DEPENDENT TYPE

The dependent personality type puts forth great effort to avoid seeming hostile, independent, or powerful (Level I). Dependent types work hard at being agreeable, willing participants, and helpful. They frequently state their preferences for not being in charge or having to make decisions that might affect others (Level II). This type has discovered that anxiety can be most effectively dealt with by relying upon others for guidance and direction. The person who behaves as though they are in need of leadership trains other persons to provide help and advice. By appearing weak and friendly, the dependent type thus provokes others to appear strong and friendly. Friendliness associated with weakness sends the message that one's dependence is not intended as a threat or imposition, but as the hope another will take on the leadership role without resentment. Dependent types may find military service appealing in the same way as hypernormals, but for different reasons. The hypernormal is driven by a sense of duty and the military provides a socially accepted outlet for its expression. The dependent type enjoys the structure provided by a chain of command but will be less eager to seek command themselves.

The psychological pressure exerted by the dependent's resistance to Level III is channeled into phobias, generalized anxiety, and such physical symptoms as tension, insomnia, and gastrointestinal distress. The latter especially communicate "a helpless, uncertain, frightened, hopeful, dependent passivity."[20] At Level III, dependant types tend to reveal a surprising elitist quality. For example, the dependant will gladly stand back and allow someone else to take on the mantle of authority and yet, comment privately, "I wouldn't waste my time taking on that much responsibility. If s/he thinks they're so smart, let them do it!" When confronted with what they've said, the dependant denies any critical intention and quickly becomes affable and compliant. Their elitism is a defense against the independence and risk to self-esteem that they associate with being in the public eye.

Just like the overlyconventional, dependent types experience much intrapersonal ambivalence about Level III traits. It is as though they sense there is something socially unacceptable lurking within and if they yield to its expression, they will be rejected by others, and if this occurs, they will have to function independently. In a sense, it is as though they would prefer to be invisible than have to take the risks associated with performing without support.

It might be tempting to imagine dependent types as good candidates for therapy because of their desire to be in a relationship that supplies guidance, direction, and support. The truth is, as long as the therapist refrains from exploring the personality too deeply, the dependent does, indeed, tend to remain in therapy. However, we do the patient no favors by restricting our attention to Level I and Level II character traits. Doing so may actually reinforce the patient's symptomology with the result that therapy deteriorates into a chat session with no visible changes taking place in the patient. If the therapist proceeds deeper into the patient's psyche, the distrust and isolation that lie at Level III will emerge and the patient will drop out of therapy to avoid the anxiety that accompanies the threat to his or her defensive system. Accordingly, long term we tend to see poor outcomes with the dependent type.

There is another important factor to consider when dealing with the dependent type and that is their proclivity for phobic symptoms. According to Leary, the "fears of the phobic are, in essence, displaced fears . . . the relatively innocuous stimuli avoided by these patients generally stand for more directly intimate interpersonal figures who are covertly feared . . . (this allows) the patient to preserve a consciously conforming, docile relationship with close figures against whom he may feel negative, rebellious emotions."[21] Fear can be externalized (fear of animals, open spaces, etc.) or it may be internalized and displaced onto the body. When fears are internalized, they find expression in physical symptoms that allow the patient to maintain a self-image as a helpless, depressed, anxious individual in need of help. Interestingly, hypochondriacal complaints may also have dependent overtones. In any case, the patient suffering from various diffuse physical symptoms rarely complains about the interpersonal issues that lie at the heart of the problems. Instead, they displace or transfer their anxiety to various parts of the body, thus distancing themselves from psychological distress. Accordingly, when we see internalized fear and its consequent physical symptomology, what we're really seeing is somatization in the dependent type. Furthermore, because phobic symptoms usually have an enduring quality, we are more likely to see chronic somatization in the dependent personality.

Because phobias may serve as a defense against anxiety, dependent types are actually somewhat less likely to become pure somatizers. Counterintuitive as this may sound, it means the presence of a phobia protects the patient from exploring an anxiety-provoking situation. Once these individuals begin feeling better in the course of therapy, we may see a flight into health as the patient unconsciously tries to avoid further therapeutic examination. Working with hysteric-phobic patients is problematic for therapists because, while we tend to examine our own emotional responses as well as the patient's, hysteric-phobics avoid self-examination as the result of their solidly entrenched repression of Level III traits.

If one observes a high degree of obsessiveness along with the hysteric-phobic qualities, we find we are dealing with a body-scanner, someone who is constantly looking for a perceived illness. If a hysteric-phobic has a long history of chronic illness complaints, his or her personality will have lost much of its resiliency. We call this condition a "fixed pathological state," out of which it is extraordinarily difficult to dislodge a patient. On the one hand, they can't improve and on the other, they can't grow worse. They have found a level of functioning that is somehow workable and they are loath to abandon it. If a patient decompensates rapidly, clinical wisdom states s/he will tend to recover rapidly; the longer it takes for a patient's defenses to break down, the harder it is for them to recover and the more likely they are to form a fixed pathological state.

THE MANAGERIAL-AUTOCRATIC TYPE

The managerial-autocratic type is characterized at Level I by "compulsive energy, authority, and dominance over others."[22] These individuals express strength and leadership qualities, seeking to win respect and admiration. Independence and competence are highly prized (Level II). Strength, however, is not merely a physical attribute, and the managerial type may seek respect through educational achievement. Prestige and financial success can also express the power drive of the managerial type. Because leaders need followers, wherever one finds the managerial type, the dependent type is sure to be present as well. On the negative side, managerial types may seem domineering, power-ridden, and overambitious, traits which reflect their own multilevel ambivalence about dependence and failure. For example, among medical residents we observe an appropriate motivation to develop competence and skill. However, the resident who is caught up in avoidance of Level III traits may have a great deal of difficulty admitting a lack of expertise in situations where consulting with their supervising physician would be appropriate. The development of maturity in the managerial type resident involves overcoming ambivalence about asking for help. In situations where a more empathetic and flexible approach to persons might be appropriate, the managerial type is often inclined to maintain the façade of authority and efficiency. In addition, the managerial type's desire to impress others may backfire when individuals who are truly accomplished regard the excessive claims of the managerial type as boring and egocentric. Psychosomatic symptoms and addictive behaviors are the most common complaints that bring the managerial type to the clinic.

Because the compulsive managerial type appears so intent on being competent, capable, and independent, it might be imagined he or she would fare somewhat better in treatment than the other types, but when we examine the multilevel pattern, the picture doesn't look much better. At the symptomatic level, the managerial group stresses responsibility and conventional strength. They do not readily admit experiencing emotional symptoms and tend to manifest bland hypernormal behavior. In their conscious, Level II self-descriptions, they emphasize toughness and self-confidence. However, in their preconscious, Level III imagery, a marked conflict appears and they express passivity and dependence. Their total personality pattern reveals an enormous interlevel variability with conflict observed between overt responsible independence and covert passivity.

Analytical and nonanalytical writers alike have emphasized the passive-dependence which underlies the energetic, success-oriented traits overtly claimed by managerial types. The combination of independence and passivity usually indicates a poor treatment motivation as well as an inclination to deny the very need for treatment. Essentially too proud to ask for help, managerial types have a mixed prognosis because they inevitably undergo a measure of personality disorganization as their public façade melts and depressive, fearful dependency emerges.

As is observed with the hypernormal, it is not only difficult to get the managerial type into therapy, but it is even more difficult to terminate therapy with them once their defensive posture toward treatment has disintegrated. So powerful are their dependency issues that, once activated, the patient may regress to an earlier stage of emotional development with the therapist consequently taking on the role of parent. For this reason alone, the clinician must be judicious when probing the managerial's unconscious. Unless s/he is fully prepared to support the patient through the entire process of resolving his or her regression, it may be better to either transfer the patient or simply leave well enough alone. Unless you have something better to offer the patient, don't tear down their defenses needlessly.

Years ago, the managerial type was referred to as the "ulcer" personality since these individuals were regarded as prototypical for experiencing gastrointestinal problems. Prior to the discovery of *H. pylori*, the etiology of stomach ulcers was considered psychosomatic. Nevertheless, despite the availability of pharmacological treatment for gastric ulcers (histamine blockers, proton pump inhibitors, and antibiotics), there remains some utility in identifying psychosomatic elements in ulcer patients. One might say that pharmacology has produced a medical defense system against the need for psychological therapy. The ulcer, which has gotten out of control, places the patient squarely in a psychosomatic framework, but since drugs can resolve the symptoms, we are less inclined to examine them psychologically. As with the hysterical patients of the early days of Freud, Janet, and Charcot, which have come to be regarded in our present culture as possessing characterological disorders rather than hysterical neuroses, ulcer patients are still psychosomatic but now we see them as somatizers. Pharmacology masks the outward psychosomatic ulcer. This is called altering the form of the symptom to adapt to changing therapeutic developments. Today's chronic fatigue syndrome is yesterday's neurasthenia; yesterday's ulcer is today's somatizing syndrome.

THE COMMON ELEMENT

The common element between these four personality types would seem to be their mutual fear of the eruption of Level III contents into consciousness resulting in the progressive disorganization we discussed in chapter 4. When ego structures progressively break down, Level III material intrudes into conscious experience generating a host of interpersonal difficulties. But there is more to the picture because Leary's Interpersonal Checklist reveals variability at each level. For example, a hypernormal should be expected to demonstrate some kind of power orientation; the closer they are to the managerial-autocratic type, the greater the need to express power and mastery, albeit in a socially acceptable manner. When Level III traits begin to appear at Level I, they are often heralded at Level II by suspiciousness, hostility, and social withdrawal. Patients will complain of being misunderstood, abused, or unappreciated. We note this phenomenon particularly among somatizing patients whose preconscious fantasies reveal ideas associated with being weary, torn, unloved, and experiencing a barren existence.

At the same time, somatizers generally show skeptical, distrustful, suspicious, and hostile traits that are associated with the paranoid vector of the circumplex. Initially, this may seem confusing to the reader, so let us explain what we mean. Level III traits are identified by a reciprocal conflict relationship with the personality type 180 degrees opposite the one we're examining:

Overlyconventional—Sadistic
Hypernormal—Rebellious
Managerial-Autocratic—Masochistic
Competitive-Narcissistic—Dependent

When we begin to see Level III traits manifested in the patient, we know our relationship has changed and we need to adjust our expectations accordingly. Sadistic personalities tend to be cruel, self-centered, manipulative, and lack empathy for other individuals. From the perspective of the DSM-IV-TR, we'd diagnosis them with Antisocial Personality Disorder. When these traits are manifested in the overlyconventional, we see anger, resentment, and demanding, vengeful behaviors. Rebelliousness is connected with disregard for social norms, odd or unusual attire, risk-taking, and nonconformity. Masochism describes harm avoidance and these personalities strive to send the message, "I'm harmless, don't hurt me." Competitive-Narcissistic types are self-interested, competitive, and extremely image conscious.

When individuals show Level III scores that lie close to masochism or rebelliousness, these traits complicate the Level III picture. Instead of a "pure"

Level III, we see traits that seem more paranoid and defensive in nature. In other words, instead of a hypernormal merely fantasizing about abandoning job and family to become a stand-up comedian, they begin to act out. When the somatizing hypernormal perceives a threat to his or her character structure, in the form of psychological probing or the clinician's ambivalence, Level III paranoid masochism is activated. Such persons complain of being misunderstood, misdiagnosed, and show signs of suspiciousness, mistrust, and covert hostility. Obsessive qualities and phobic behavior become more pronounced and patients seem even more withdrawn and disconnected from the clinician. What we're seeing is the rubric of helplessness that becomes fixated into the body system. Fear and mistrust provoke angry behavior that acts as a detaching mechanism to eliminate anxiety and justify the patient's preconceptions.

Leary's discussion of the psychotic personality is revealing in this context. Generally, psychotic types are prone to deny symptoms and present as strong, healthy persons. Their self-report emphasizes conventional normality and they claim a "pious sweetness and cooperative sociability."[23] At Level II, therefore, we see traits consistent with the four personality types described above. In contrast to our contemporary definitions of psychosis involving hallucinations, ideas of reference, delusions, and the like, Leary is talking about character structure.

> Psychosis . . . is related in many cases to a desperate attempt to maintain a normal, conventional, innocent façade in teeth of deeper feelings of weakness and worthlessness. In other cases, psychosis is characterized by a solid multi-level structure of despair and distrust. . . . Whenever a patient presents a multilevel pattern which involves claimed conventional friendliness contrasted with a distrustful or masochistic Level III score, the danger flag should be flown. This is the paranoid phenomenon.[24]

While these individuals adhere to socially accepted norms at Level II, at Level I we observe reticence and guardedness, especially in treatment. When the clinician seems uncertain, withholding, or attempts to engage in therapeutic probing, Level III paranoid masochism is activated and the relationship breaks down. Clinicians may find themselves on the receiving end of the dependant type's narcissistic passive aggression, the hypernormal's angry mistrust, and so forth. Whatever combination of traits is activated, the driving force seems very similar to Leary's paranoid phenomenon.

At the deepest levels, among hypernormals, overlyconventionals, managerial-autocratics, and dependant types who utilize somatization, the common element is more than a fear of progressive personality deterioration: it is the presence of paranoid masochism at Level III. The reciprocal conflict between culturally identified values at Level II and Level III traits combined with paranoid masochism results in multilevel ambivalence and reinforces the process of somatization.

AVOIDING IMPASSE RESISTANCE

We said earlier that the clinician's perception and experience of the patient represents a combination of listening and observation. We listen to the patient's self-report as well as his responses to our questions and observe his behavior. While Level III may creep into his comments during the initial session(s), his behavior reveals far more. Impasse resistance develops when we focus on the self-report and overlook Level III. The most effective way of managing impasse resistance is to avoid it in the first place. This is accomplished by learning to cooperate with the patient's real intention, rather than his stated one. With somatizing patients, this means recognizing that, while the patient states he wants relief from their symptoms, his behavior over time indicates a strong attachment to them and efforts to eliminate them will be met with resistance.

The dynamic interplay between Levels II and III can make working with somatizing patients a perplexing experience. Clinicians are accustomed to assuming patients mean what they say when they insist they are weary of being in pain, feeling socially isolated, depressed, and so forth. We attempt to establish treatment goals by inquiring, for instance, "What do you think is the most important thing we can fix today?" Somatizing patients tell us what they believe to be their primary concerns, but their behavior says otherwise. For example, a patient's history indicates a series of failed treatments and unsatisfactory relationships with other medical practitioners. We initiate treatment directed at symptomatic reduction and within a matter of days, the patient reports she isn't feeling any better and doesn't believe she can continue the current medication. We decide to change dosing strategies or begin a trial of another medication. Despite feeling initially optimistic, only a short time passes before the patient reports the medication "isn't working." This pattern continues for several weeks until either doctor, patient, or both become frustrated with the lack of progress. Our best efforts notwithstanding, we begin to form the impression that the patient is intent on defeating any treatment we prescribe. And the fact is, our impression is correct.

Somatization is a powerful defensive strategy and a patient's unconscious attachment to it can be equally powerful. So powerful, in fact, that the clinician's efforts to help the patient can be perceived as a threat to ego integrity. In such a situation, the patient has little choice but to try to eliminate the threat and this is accomplished by defeating the clinician. Patients achieve this aim by setting a trap for the clinician.[25] This occurs when the clinician mistakes the patient's Level II report for their actual intention. The trap is sprung when the clinician endeavors to treat the Level II concern.[26] Eventually patient and doctor are at odds with one another, the relationship crumbles, treatment failure ensues, and the patient moves on to another clinician.

We avoid impasse resistance by aligning ourselves with the patient's Level III intentionality. In the case of somatization, this means we admit to the patient that her condition eludes diagnosis given the present state of medical science. However, we go on to explain that we can assist her by helping her learn how to better manage her symptoms. We stress the importance of learning effective coping skills, tracking symptom severity, and working together as members of a treatment team. We urge her to begin Cognitive-Behavioral or Dialectical Behavioral Therapy and explain how the mind can be an extremely valuable tool for reducing anxiety. We express support for her illness beliefs and arrange for regularly spaced follow-up appointments. Our long-term goals include establishing a stable working relationship with such a patient, helping her feel more empowered within the limits set by her personality organization, and assisting her in her efforts to preserve ego integrity without compromising medical care.

It is tempting to follow Alfred Adler's suggestion that we reframe the patient's self-report, that is, "You've said you want to get better, but you seem to have difficulty with the medications we are trying."[27] Comments like this interpret the patient's resistance and are intended to bring it into conscious perception. Individuals with a healthy ego can use this information appropriately to see how they are to a certain extent responsible for their response to treatment. In the case of chronic somatizing patients, however, any indication that we believe they are clinging to their symptoms results in vehement denial. Level III intentions are as unconscious as somatization. Our very best "treatment" may be to help these patients consciously accept their illness and learn to rely on more effective skills for managing life stressors.

CONCLUDING THOUGHTS

By now it should be obvious that one should not merely assign somatizing patients to psychotherapy as a matter of routine. The presence of Level III traits in the overlyconventional, dependent, hypernormal, and managerial-autocratic personality types and their purposefully constructed patterns of defense render it necessary to engage in careful screening as part of any treatment plan. Furthermore, even when a course of therapy is indicated, the clinician must proceed with caution. When working with pre-psychotic anger and resentment, the clinician must move forward slowly and deliberately, and avoid withdrawing support from the patient. Eagerness to see results may prompt either the patient's premature withdrawal from therapy or even facilitate the decompensation against which the patient is so strongly defended. In some situations, the patient lacks sufficient ego strength to cope with the slightest degree of exploration by the therapist and should be given the opportunity to "repress out" of therapy or be seen for supportive therapy alone. In any case, the task of the clinician is to be sensitive to pressure from the patient to withdraw from probing, and support the anxiety, depression, or obsessive solutions to which the patient may turn for relief. Even with those patients who seem to possess the ability to endure the self-examination inherent in therapy, the clinician should not only monitor the patient for signs of anxiety which mark the limits of their ability to tolerate conscious awareness of underlying feelings, but also be alert for psychotic trends or a flight into health. In addition, the clinician must remember that, while multilevel patterns of personality may differ somewhat between the various types, when established early in the treatment planning phase, these patterns are extremely valuable for predicting a patient's prognosis.

Because the evaluation of personality involves serious consideration of the interplay between the levels of personality, the potential for somatization will vary with ego integrity or stability. Certainly, the therapist's observations of the patient as well as the patient's self-report yield valuable information concerning personality type as it relates to somatization. But it does not follow that somatization is a necessary corollary of personality type. If this were true, the number of cases would be huge, equal to the number of overlyconventionals and the other personality types discussed herein in the population. What should be considered is how interlevel variability can account for degrees of severity present in somatization. Studies of personality type are not intended to provide a diagnostic shortcut; rather they function to enable the practitioner to more fully understand the difficulties involved in identifying and treating the somatizing patient. Somatizers are highly conventional people and their heightened ambivalence is often revealed beneath the functional, albeit defensive, public façade. When a patient's Level I and Level II presentation begins to crumble in the face of overwhelming anxiety, the body becomes the final line of defense which, in the patient's mind, is absolute, inviolable, and impenetrable. Armed with Level III information in advance, we know more fully what to expect and how to anticipate interpersonal difficulties with those people prone to somatization. It falls to the clinician, utilizing the tools presented in the following chapters, to be a source of positive support and help to these patients, rather than allowing relationships with them to deteriorate into just one more experience of failure and despair.

Chapter Seven

Cognitive Behavioral Treatments of Chronic Somatization

One of the most frequent questions encountered among clinicians is, how do we approach the chronic somatizer with an effective therapy? Typically, insight-oriented psychotherapy is a less than optimal approach. Few somatizing patients possess the psychological mindedness and motivation to undergo the kind of in-depth analysis that takes place in psychodynamic therapy.

At some point, the underlying issues involved in somatization will have to be addressed and this involves therapeutic probing, and probing, more often than not, results in an increase in somatization, slowing the process of therapy. Guthrie describes some success with a short-term dynamic model in the treatment of irritable bowel syndrome, suggesting possible applicability of this approach with other functional somatic syndromes.[1] For most patients, however, symptom management is the priority and behavioral therapies are far better suited for this purpose.

How can we help chronic somatizers manage their "disability" and live more functional lives? Studies suggest the usefulness of Cognitive Behavioral Therapy (CBT) for the treatment of patients with diagnosed somatoform disorders.[2] We think this is, without question, a wise approach. We know all too well that we are neither going to change nor cure the chronic somatizer. Rather than challenge their perceptions, we choose to work *with* them. Instead of allowing the patient to restrict themselves to the role of the "sick person," we enlist them as real members of the treatment team by teaching them to manage their symptoms.

Before we begin our discussion, however, a word of explanation is indicated. There are a number of therapies that are commonly subsumed under the general rubric of "cognitive behavior therapy," including Rational-Emotive Therapy, Dialectical Behavior Therapy (reviewed in the next chapter), cognitive therapy, coping skills training, problem-solving therapies, self-instructional training, and self-control approaches.[3] While there are some differences in the theoretical bases, the strategies for implementation, and the like, of these approaches, there are also similarities: They are usually time limited and structured, and assume that affect and behavior result from ways in which the patient construes the world.[4] The function of therapy is to enable the patient to identify, reality test, and correct maladaptive conceptualizations and beliefs.[5] For our purposes, CBT (also "standard CBT") refers to the model of therapy associated with the work of Aaron Beck.[6] In addition, we shall examine the potential use of Cognitive-Behavioral Modification Therapy as developed by Donald Meichenbaum.

COGNITIVE BEHAVIOR THERAPY

Generally speaking, CBT asserts that the way individuals interpret their experience determines how they feel and behave.[7] Reality-based interpretations result in situation-congruent feelings and manageable behaviors. Interpretations derived from biased information yields distortions in perception that result in distressing emotions and behaviors that may be maladaptive. Our responses to experience are thus highly individualized; what is troublesome to one is hardly noticeable to another. What predisposes an individual to experience psychological distress is the interplay between factors such as childhood experiences, personality differences, and developmental history: "The match between a person's specific vulnerability (e.g., sees herself as worthless unless she is loved) and a significant life event that reflects this intermediate belief (e.g., she becomes depressed after her partner rejects her) is likened . . . to a key fitting into a lock or, technically speaking, a stress-diathesis model where the stress is adverse life events (precipitating factors) and the diathesis is the cognitive vulnerability (predisposing factors)."[8]

Two key elements figure into the process of interpretation and response; that is, schemas (also known as core beliefs or basic assumptions) and automatic thoughts. Schemas tend to come about as the result of early learning experiences and may reflect positively on the individual (e.g., "I'm popular") or negatively (e.g., "I've never been a popular person"). Schemas serve as a means of processing incoming information and "determine how we perceive events; in a sense, we can only see what the core belief allows us to. Dormant negative core beliefs are often activated and thereby pass into our awareness at times of emotional distress."[9] CBT posits that certain individuals are predisposed to psychopathology in large measure because of these schemas, which may become enduring cognitive patterns within a personality structure. According to Beck et al.:

> Although different persons may conceptualize the same situation in different ways, a particular person tends to be consistent in his responses to similar types of events. Relatively stable cognitive patterns form the basis for the regularity of interpretations of a particular set of situations. . . . When a person faces a particular circumstance, a schema related to the circumstance is activated. The schema is the basis for molding data into cognitions. . . . Thus, a schema constitutes the basis for screening out, differentiating, and coding the stimuli that confront the individual. He categorizes and evaluates his experience through a matrix of schemas.[10]

In psychopathological conditions such as depression or anxiety, individuals construct interpretations of their experience according to a set of defective schemas. In milder cases of pathology, persons may retain some ability to view their experience objectively; in more severe cases, objectivity becomes increasingly difficult to maintain, and cognitions may become completely dominated by schemas that promote negative thinking, ruminations, perseveration, and the like.[11]

Automatic thoughts are interpretations of experience that occur rapidly, often at the edge of consciousness, and may include specific verbal ideas and images.[12] Frequently congruent with the emotion one is experiencing, automatic thoughts seem completely believable, accurate renditions of what is taking place. Thus, automatic thoughts reinforce one's emotions and, in retrospect, often provide justification for consequent behavior. A simplified model of the way in which events, schemas, and automatic thoughts influence emotions and behavior is shown in figure 7.1.[13]

Environmental stimuli (events) trigger cognitive processes (schema and automatic thoughts) which give the event personal meaning, resulting in behavioral and emotional symptoms.[14] The two-way arrows between behavioral and emotional symptoms and automatic thoughts indicate these are mutually reinforcing. An automatic thought interpreting an event as beyond an individual's coping capacity generates anxiety and social withdrawal which, in turn, generate additional automatic thoughts reinforcing the individual's original perception, thus generating increased anxiety and a desire to avoid the initial stimulus.

CBT posits several patterns of irrational thinking that can result in cognitive distortions or negative automatic thoughts.[15]

- Overgeneralization—drawing general conclusions across all situations based on a single event.

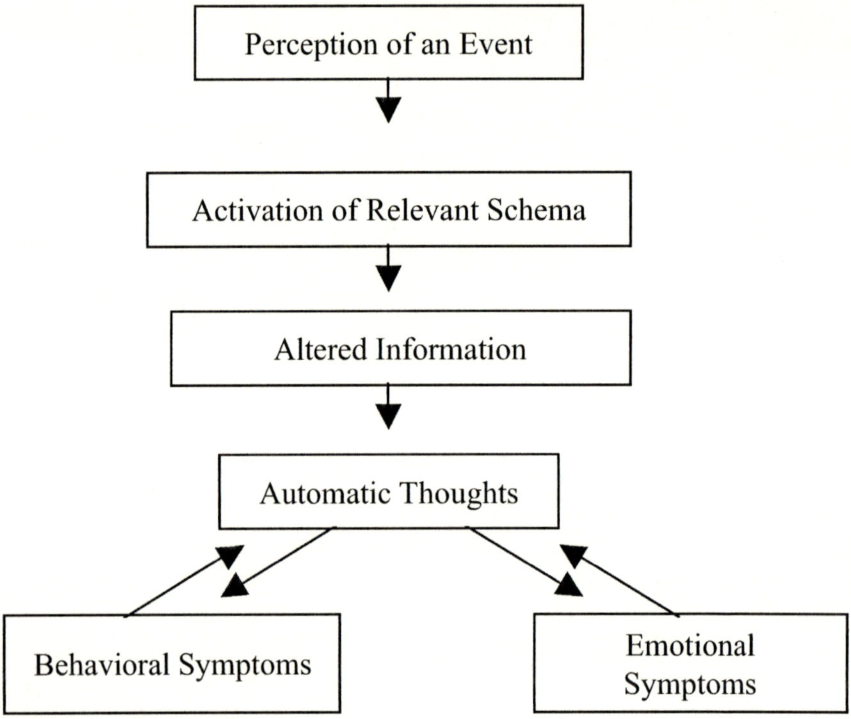

Figure 7.1

- Personalization—the inclination to attribute personal significance to events even in the face of contradicting evidence.
- Maximizing and minimizing—distorted evaluation of the relative importance of particular events.
- Selective abstraction—focusing on a detail taken out of context, ignoring other, valid features of the situation, and conceptualizing the whole on the basis of this single detail.
- Dichotomous (all-or-nothing) thinking—the tendency to view events in black and white terms.
- Arbitrary inference—drawing a conclusion in the absence of supporting evidence or even in the face of contradictory evidence.

One of the primary goals of CBT is to teach the patient ways of countering his or her typical cognitive distortions in order to interpret the experience in ways that reflect a more realistic here and now perspective, reducing emotional distress and enabling more functional behavior. In this model, the therapist assumes the role of an empathetic teacher who engages the patient in a collaborative relationship in which the patient's cognitive assumptions can be reframed into a testable hypothesis. Together, therapist and patient engage in reality testing of the patient's automatic thoughts and assumptions. As the treatment progresses, the focus eventually turns to evaluating the patient's underlying schemas in the same way as automatic thoughts; namely, in terms of their supporting evidence, their logical basis, and empirical testing. Reading and homework assignments are also techniques employed by cognitive therapists. Homework assignments may proceed on graded levels, from simple to more complex and demanding, enabling patients to practice reframing automatic thoughts in real life settings. Homework is reviewed in therapy where problems and resistance are evaluated with a view to improving future performance.

An important starting point for the application of CBT to functional somatic syndromes is the observation that these individuals demonstrate similarities to depressive and anxious populations, with whom CBT has been extensively researched. To begin with, depressed persons tend to reflect a negative view of themselves, their interpersonal environment, and their outlook on life.[16] Anxious individuals tend to make fearful predictions of their performance under stress or their relationships with others.[17] The difficulty with this kind of thinking is not solely its negative focus, but the fact that it tends to be self-perpetuating. Underlying schemas motivate individuals to use, for instance, selective abstraction with the result that they undervalue their capabilities, ignore their successes, or focus on their failures. In our experience, individuals with somatizing or functional somatic syndromes often think in similar fashion. They may hold irrational or uninformed beliefs about the nature of illness as well as the meaning of bodily sensations. According to Taerk:

> Central to cognitive theory is the view that a patient's cognitions are of primary importance in determining his or her behavior and his or her emotional and physiological state. Patients with functional somatic symptoms commonly hold dysfunctional beliefs. Just as the thinking of patients suffering from depressive disorders is typically dysfunctional in that it tends to a distorted and excessively negative view of the self, the world, and the future, patients with functional somatic syndromes commonly hold similar beliefs concerning their physical health and functioning. They tend to attribute bodily sensations to physical disease rather than to emotional or trivial causes.[18]

The beliefs that somatizing patients maintain about the nature of illness and bodily sensations can be a great source of health anxiety. According to Salkovskis, when symptoms are perceived as a threat, autonomic responses become more pronounced and these are then interpreted by the patient as further evidence of illness.[19] Even normal variations in body functions may be perceived by somatizing patients as representing some change from their baseline experience, from which the conclusion is drawn that these changes are pathological.[20] Robbins and Kirmayer draw attention to the term "somatosensory amplification" as "the tendency to experience somatic sensations as intense, noxious, or disturbing."[21] As a result of these misperceptions of physical experience and the attending increase in anxiety, patients may engage in avoidance behaviors intended to reduce illness anxiety. Social withdrawal, cessation of pleasurable activities, and discontinuance of exercise regimens are common examples of avoidance behaviors. Ironically, the effect may be just the opposite of what was intended. Individuals who cease exercising, for example, find their energy levels decrease and, rather than accurately attributing this to reduced activity, determine the loss of energy as confirmation of their illness perceptions. Avoidance behaviors "sustain symptoms by decreasing activity tolerance and increasing sensitivity to any stimulation . . . (the) result is a vicious circle of symptoms, avoidance, fatigue, demoralization, and depression."[22]

Interpersonal factors may figure largely in the perpetuation of disease preoccupation. The comments of family, friends, and even health professionals can be anxiety provoking and inadvertently reinforce the patient's insistence that s/he is actually seriously ill. Patients' beliefs about illness can create a confirmatory bias regarding disease-related information such that they selectively notice and recall experiences that are consistent with their beliefs. Even well-intentioned comments by physicians, therapists, and other medical professionals, may be taken by the patient as evidence that, "she's just trying to be gentle with me; it's just as I feared."

CBT can take place in both individual and group contexts, and each has its advantages. Individual therapy allows the patient to feel his or her concerns are important enough to warrant personal attention. In addition, since interpersonal relationships tend to be difficult for somatizing patients, individual therapy may allow more time to develop a therapeutic alliance. Some patients may feel uncomfortable in a group setting; in this case individual therapy is a better match. Group therapy gives the patient an opportunity to derive support and obtain feedback from other members. In dynamic terms, the group may come to serve as an auxiliary ego for some patients, and thus promote compliance. Furthermore, teaching CBT concepts may seem less threatening in a group context; instead of taking on the atmosphere of "therapy," the group seems more like a classroom in which coping skills are presented. In both settings, homework assignments are important treatment elements and may include monitoring symptoms and recording automatic thoughts. Symptom checklists enable patients to identify the conditions under which symptoms seem more noticeable and whether a particular skill was useful in reducing symptom severity. The same holds true for automatic thoughts; by recording automatic thoughts, patients can become more aware of the messages they send themselves and the ways in which their automatic thoughts generate stress, anxiety, and the like.

The key element in CBT is the communication of empathy. Mindful of the somatizing patient's sensitivity to suggestions that his condition reflects psychological factors, the therapist must be very careful to reassure the patient that his symptoms are taken seriously. CBT aims at empowering patients to develop a sense of capability in the management of their symptoms. Even following a course of individual or group CBT therapy, patients may still cling to the hope that their physical problems belie the presence of a physical disease—and, indeed, this may be true. As the senior author pointed out in chapter 2, today's somatizing syndrome may be tomorrow's yet-to-be-defined illness. Even if this proves not to be the case, the patient's hope informs us that he or she is aware, doubtless quite unconsciously, that somatization meets a need that even the best therapy cannot. Accordingly, the goal of CBT with the chronic population is symptom reduction, not the elimination of somatization. If patients report lower symptom frequency, fewer doctor visits, less reliance on analgesic medications, and a higher, more satisfying quality of life, we've accomplished our task quite neatly.

COGNITIVE BEHAVIORAL MODIFICATION THERAPY

CBT is conceptualized on the basis of an information-processing model that stresses that patients' cognitive errors about the nature of the experience of reality reflect cognitive schemas, current issues, and basic assumptions brought to real-life situations.[23] As noted above, patients are depressed, for example, because they distort the nature of reality as a result of cognitive errors and irrational beliefs. Useful as the information processing model may be, it is also possible to utilize a constructivist perspective for conceptualizing the ways in which patients construct their personal realities and create representational models of the world.[24]

> [Following a constructivist model] the human mind is a product of constructive symbolic activity, and that reality is a product of personal meanings that individuals create. It is not as if there is one reality and clients distort that reality, thus contributing to their problems; rather, there are multiple realities, and the task for the therapist is to help clients become aware of how they create these realities and of the consequences of such constructions.[25]

The constructivist model is represented in Cognitive Behavior Modification Therapy (CBMT), developed by Donald Meichenbaum.

One practical expression of constructivism in CBMT is the application of Narrative Therapy (NT) in its approach.[26] According to NT, individuals attempt to make sense of personal history by connecting events in a narrative or story. Meaning-making is an important aspect of human experience, especially insofar as it involves the creation of symbols. In myth, literature, and religion, for example, elements of human and nonhuman experience are interwoven in ways that take on individual, societal, and/or cultural significance. Similarly, following narrative therapy, patients tell and retell the tale of their lives, incorporating new experiences and interpreting them in the light of previous experience and the overall plot line. A basic premise of CBMT is that generation of such narrative explanations is an essentially adaptive response.[27] Unlike standard CBT that posits a patient's history tends to be interlaced with maladaptive schemas and cognitive distortions, CBMT recognizes that elements of the patient's narrative account represent the attempt to make sense of very difficult and painful experiences. What becomes problematic about these efforts is the tendency of patients to become "stuck" and view their personal narrative as the *only* possible one. According to the constructivist metaphor, the role of the therapist is to act as a co-constructivist, listening "empathetically and reflectively to the initial story line of the patient and then collaboratively help the client transform his or her story."[28]

In the initial stage of therapy, one validates the patient's efforts, making comments such as, "Don't you think anyone would feel much as you do, under these circumstances?" No effort is made at this point to offer corrections to the patient's ways of thinking or their conceptualizations of their history. Establishment of a cooperative, collaborative therapeutic relationship is critical; Meichenbaum calls it the "glue" that makes the other elements of CBMT work.[29]

> You need to encourage clients to tell their stories, at their own pace and to be in charge. Be out of the telling of their stories, out of the narrative sharing—and there's a lot of therapeutic value in sharing one's story—new stories emerge that also reveal strengths and resources. Clients' stories are filled with expressions of hopelessness and helplessness. They often convey a tale of having been "victimized" and it is my job, as the therapist, not only to hear their stories and empathize with them, but also to help them appreciate what they have done to survive and to cope with their feelings, namely, help them attend to the "rest of the story." For the "rest of the story" is often a tale of remarkable strengths. Keep in mind that the story of how people cope with stressful events is inherently the story of resilience and courage. . . . Thus, the "bad things" that happened to people are only one chapter in their life stories.[30]

Principles that Meichenbaum borrows from psychodynamic theory are (1) following the patient's affect and (2) affirming the value of the corrective emotional experience.[31] With regard to the first principle, patient comments that are affect-laden are pointed out by the therapist for particular attention, since emotion serves as an indicator of important elements in the narrative. Concerning the second, meaningful change is affect-laden. In CBMT, we aren't trying to secure a purely intellectual acceptance of certain kinds of data nor do we assume that patients will be convinced simply because the data indicates one thing or another. We want them to actively use the data to alter their beliefs and create for themselves a more adaptive and health-affirming inner dialogue.

An interesting distinction between CPT and CBMT lies in what we might call "meaning attribution." According to Meichenbaum, it isn't that people distort reality or make cognitive errors that contribute to their suffering, but rather their propensity to assume there is a single reality which explains their condition.[32] The fact that a story can be told at all implies that it can be told in different ways. A series of events that seem traumatic to one individual may seem scarcely worthy of note to another. Much depends on the ways in which we describe our history, the words we choose, and the affects we experience. Learning to reconceptualize one's narrative isn't an easy task; patients construe the nature of their experience in ways they find reasonable, coherent with their understanding about the way life "works," and consistent with their personal histories; that is, what they've learned, been taught, and what has seemed true to them as matters of fact. It is important to help patients understand how their self-talk may represent the voices of a number of different influences and not their own unique "voice." From a constructivist perspective, it isn't the symptoms of psychiatric illness that impairs patients' functioning as much as it is their self-talk; that is, what they say to themselves and others about the ways they respond to situations.[33] One might be tempted to equate self-talk with the automatic thought of CBT but the difference is, self-talk represents the stories that patients tell themselves and the *meaning* they assign to their ability or lack of ability to manage life circumstances. Self-talk is not simply reactive; it represents a goal-directed, constructive process.

The task of the CBMT therapist is to help patients move away from a "deficit" model of functioning where they repeat messages of self-abasement, and learn to cognitively reframe their experiences.[34] However, we aren't referring to cognitive reframing in the sense that we wish patients to counter irrational thoughts that spring from distorted core schemas. The alternative narrative that therapist and patient work together to construct must be coherent, fit the patient's present circumstances, and be adequate in capturing and explaining his or her difficulties.[36] A patient's narrative may contain a number of coping elements that perpetuate rather than ameliorate pain and distress, but it represents the patient's best understanding of reality. Alternative narratives must be equally viable or the patient will find them unacceptable. Part of what we wish patients to realize is, what matters most about narrative construction is not the historical truthfulness of the narrative, but its narrative truthfulness.[37] Even the patient's initial story may be factually incongruent with what actually has occurred; in some cases, historical verification of the events of the narrative may be impossible. For example, key players may be dead or inaccessible in some other way. What makes the narrative "work" for the patient is the meaning s/he assigns to it; alternative narratives must communicate a similar sense of plausibility in order for the patient to embrace them as meaningful.

CBMT is a behavioral therapy and this means that translation of the patient's narrative from the deficit model to the more self-affirming one that is coauthored by patient and therapist eventually embraces behavioral change. Meichenbaum's strategy at this point involves, first, eliciting an inventory of patient strengths; second, asking an "in spite of" question; and concluding with a "how" question.[38] Identification of character strengths helps identify coping resources of which the patient may be unaware and which may be capitalized upon to foster a greater sense of mastery. When the patient identifies a character strength or evidence of positive coping, the question is asked, "In spite of all you have been through (give specific examples), you were able to do such and such?" This question is followed by, "How were you able to do that? Where did you find the courage?"[39] In this way, patient and therapist explore the ways in which patients can cope effectively and incorporate credit for their changes into their self-talk.

In an earlier work, Meichenbaum suggested four guidelines for developing a skills training program:

1. Coping devices are complex and need to be flexible. Coping devices that are successful in one situation may be quite unsuccessful in another situation, or even the same situation at another time. Thus, any coping-skills training approach should be flexible enough to incorporate a variety of cognitive and behavioral strategies that can be differentially employed.
2. Consistent with the call for flexibility is the need for any training technique to be sensitive to individual differences, cultural differences, and situational differences.
3. Skills training should encourage the utilization of available information and the incorporation of potentially threatening events into cognitive plans. To be effective, information should stimulate mental rehearsal or the "work of worrying" that may "short-circuit" the experience of stress or reduce its after effects.
4. Actual exposure during training to less threatening stressful events has a beneficial effect.[40]

Adaptive coping skills allow the patient to experience the stressful events of their lives in measured doses, permitting the development of a sense of mastery that provides inoculation against greater incidences of threat.[41] Meichenbaum's own program of skills training is called Stress Inoculation Therapy (SIT) and is composed of three phases: An initial conceptualization phase, a skills acquisition and rehearsal phase, and an application and follow through phase.[42] During the first phase, a collaborative therapist-patient relationship is established in which patients are encouraged to view perceived threats as problems to be solved and to identify those situations and reactions which are amenable to change and which ones are not.[43] Over time, the patient's stress response is reconceptualized in a manner that is specific to a given patient's real-life situation and problem areas.[44] In phase two, coping skills such as self-soothing, relaxation training, problem solving, and the like are taught, practiced, and rehearsed in ways that are tailored to the specific stressors encountered by the patient.[45] Phase three focuses on skills reinforcement by practicing them along a gradient of increasing levels of stress. Patients may be asked to help other patients learn skills in order to consolidate their own skills application ("See one, do one, teach one").[46] Relapse prevention, exercises in attribution that help patients take credit for their behavioral gains, and follow-up sessions also figure into phase three.[47] SIT has been employed in the treatment of a number of situations including biofeedback training and pain management.[48] The structure of SIT is applicable to both individual and group settings.

The use of SIT in biofeedback training is of particular interest because it deals with physiological arousal and this, of course, relates to our discussion of somatization. The initial phase of treatment involves establishing the meaning attached to the patient's symptoms. Careful consideration is paid to the patient's self-talk or internal dialogue that precedes, accompanies, and follows the patient's physiological responses.[49]

> Quite often, the client's internal dialogue concerning his physiological response includes a sense of helplessness and hopelessness and an accompanying sense of absence of control. . . . It is important to appreciate this process, for one of the consequences of biofeedback treatment may be to change the client's perceptions, attributions, appraisals—his internal dialogue about his ability to control, first, his physiological response and then his cognitions, feelings, and behaviors. . . . As we discover the content of the internal dialogue, we can incorporate, anticipate, and subsume such cognitions into treatment. Insofar as the client and therapist evolve a common conceptualization of the nature of the problem and the form of treatment, the client will be motivated to participate in treatment and comply with the training demands.[50]

As noted above, according to CBMT, it isn't the experience of physiological arousal that is debilitating, as much as it is the meaning the patient attaches to it. Eventually, the patient's symptoms themselves become cues to use higher level coping skills learned in treatment.[51] Treatment proceeds by obtaining a history and making homework assignments whereby patients can monitor their experiences and generate a sense of baseline functioning, including maladaptive coping responses typically employed by the patient. The goal is to develop an increasing awareness on the part of the patient of maladaptive physiological responses and then establish some voluntary control by means of conscious effort.[52] Monitoring internal dialogue is important in order to discourage any self-talk which may interfere with this process. As noted in our discussion of SIT, we want the patient to learn a set of coping skills which can extend beyond the therapy session.

Prior to therapy, the client is likely to view his target behavior (such as a headache) as a massive, undifferentiated attack and as a sign of further deterioration, all of which engenders anxiety and contributes to a maladaptive response. As a result of biofeedback treatment, the client is more likely to view his headaches differentially, noting the tension that precedes the headaches (i.e., prodromal signs), and viewing a headache as a series of stages varying in intensity and having a time-based or situationally based parameters. The client becomes aware of how his own reactions to his problem influence the headache, by exacerbating or decreasing it. Such recognition of his symptoms is the cue or signal to employ the coping techniques he has learned in treatment.[53]

Additional reinforcement and the promotion of generalization is provided by role playing, films modeling adaptive behaviors, and/or the therapist modeling identification of physiological arousal and then using positive coping skills in its management.

An application of SIT that is of particular interest to somatization studies is in the alleviation of pain. The idea that cognitive elements can influence pain perception is not a new one; classical and Enlightenment thinkers alike have affirmed the value of using reason or imaginative distraction to alter the awareness of pain.[54] SIT, however, is not intended as a replacement for other treatment approaches to pain (biofeedback, pharmacology, etc.) but as an augmentative strategy. When dealing with somatizing patients, this is an important element to bring to their attention. By pointing out how medical treatments can be enhanced by psychological interventions, we counter objections to engaging in therapies such as SIT.

One way of formulating the application of SIT to pain control is to use the elements of the gate control theory of pain to highlight SIT's treatment elements. Accordingly, there are three components to the pain experience; that is, sensory-discriminative, motivational-affective, and cognitive-evaluative.[55]

Presuming the clinician has engaged the patient in determining the elements of the patient's "pain narrative" and identified maladaptive coping skills, the first step involves teaching the patient a number of ways of controlling sensory input including relaxation techniques and monitoring one's breathing.[56] Reminding the patient of the effectiveness of using breathing exercises during childbirth helps reinforce the believability of sensory reduction at this stage. The motivational-affective component focuses on feelings such as helplessness and hopelessness that may characterize the patient's experience of pain. At this juncture, the clinician offers a variety of other skills that have proven helpful for persons in pain including attention diversion (utilizing alternate foci of attention while experiencing pain), somatization (attending to other bodily sensations, e.g., one's breathing), and imagery manipulations (transforming the pain experience by means of imagery, e.g., goal-directed fantasy).[57] Concerning imagery manipulations, the more elaborate the image, the more effective this technique becomes; in addition, including one's pain in the image, but transforming it into something less noxious such as imagining the painful site being numbed by medication, may be helpful.[58]

Just as in biofeedback training, where coping strategies are tailored to meet a particular patient's needs, in pain management, Meichenbaum indicates offering a number of coping skills, which can be used at the patient's own discretion, may aid patients in those moments when pain is intense and the temptation to give up and resort to maladaptive coping is strong. In the cognitive-evaluative phase, it is suggested that patients learn to view the pain experience itself as composed of several stages including preparing for the painful stressor, confronting and handling the stressor, coping with one's feelings at critical moments, and self-reinforcement.[59] Involving the patient as a collaborator, as in CBMT, and developing a personalized coping repertoire helps create a sense of mastery and capability in managing pain. Admittedly, the previous discussion is derived from Meichenbaum's own description of ways in which SIT has been used with experimentally induced pain. Nevertheless, positive responses to SIT in these settings suggest real applicability in the clinic.

What we find so intriguing about CBMT/SIT is the tremendous respect paid to the patient's conceptualization of the problem as well as efforts s/he has made to cope in a functional manner. We believe this is extremely helpful in one's dealings with the somatizing patient. These individuals frequently present with a history of frustrated treatment outcomes, often quite accurate notions about the ambivalence of treatment providers, and serious doubts about their potential for improvement. They are naturally cautious and, as a result, may be labeled as unreliable historians when, in reality, they are simply trying to avoid what they have come to expect as an inevitable experience of rejection by individuals to whom they come for help. The current authors recall an important piece of advice offered during their psychotherapy training: patients want to tell their story. Of course, the advice was intended to remind us that the patient's agenda may differ significantly from the therapist's and, if we wish to make progress with our patients, we do well to practice our listening skills. Herein lies the genius of Meichenbaum's approach. While CBMT urges behavior change, it does so within a context that values and affirms not only the details of the patient's narrative, but also the patient's affect and typical coping style. While standard CBT may be a very functional treatment option for some, especially those patients with dependent personality types who long for someone to take the lead and offer them direction, there are others who struggle mightily to make sense of their experience. Referring to these functional efforts at meaning-making as evidence of irrational thinking or dysfunctional cognitive schemas may seem repetitive of early painful experiences with parental figures that were dismissive or minimized the child's distress. It does not matter that this may not be the therapist's intention; what matters is how the patient perceives and experiences the therapist's response to their story.

If we follow a standard CBT model, we're going to conceptualize somatization as a form of intellectual error based on misinformation or misinterpretation of standardized information. Either one's understanding of biological experience represents faulty presuppositions, for instance, "Pain must indicate injury or illness," or it represents the misinterpretation of incoming data, such as, "My chest pain must indicate I'm having a heart attack" (instead of gas pains or evidence of muscle strain). In the former case, the error is conceptual; in the latter, it is an error of information processing.

A structural-developmental approach to somatic concerns shows how somatization is a function of an individual's unique ways of conceptualizing experience. Writing about faith development, Fowler observes, "It is not just the *contents* of our ideas and values that differ; at various stages in our development the fundamental *patterns of operation* within our minds may be quite different." By this he means the ways in which information processing occurs will differ according to developmental stages. A child's reasoning does not represent defective adult reasoning; instead, it indicates the child has not yet developed adult reasoning capabilities. Nevertheless, this does not mean the child's reasoning is inherently faulty: "The child's thinking has its own structures. These differ qualitatively from adult structures but are nonetheless coherent and integrated."[60] He goes on to write, "One way to understand what we mean by 'structures' of thinking and valuing is to think of the operational rules or laws which the mind follows in reasoning or making judgments. These are not conscious; we are not aware of them in such a way that we could articulate them or explain them. Rather, *they are the implicit rules underlying consciousness*. They are the patterned responses that constitute our thought."[61]

From this standpoint, somatization is much more than pathology; it structures, guides, and informs the patient's conscious awareness. Following Meichenbaum, we understand this structure as the underlying theme of the somatizing patient's individual life narrative. Like the plot of a novel, somatization gives direction and coherence to the story, it carries us from beginning chapter to the resolution at the end. In its absence we have chaos or, at best, an unconnected series of vignettes that leaves us wondering where we've come from and, if anywhere, we're going. Somatization ties the narrative together and gives the teller the sense that their experience is explicable.

CBMT offers the therapist a way to interact with the patient on a collaborative level in order to establish a relationship based on mutual understanding of the patient's story. When the patient is approached thusly, the entire perspective of treatment is altered, and some therapists might find this rather difficult to accept. We are accustomed to regarding the patient's story as representative of physical illness coupled with some measure of psychopathology. If we are going to follow Meichenbaum, we have to learn to bracket our predispositions and allow ourselves to become more flexible in our own conceptions of reality. The patient's account, instead of being a dysfunctional one that needs altering, becomes one functional account among many, and our task is to enable the patient to retell the story so as to become less focused on illness and more capable of managing life effectively. Following CBMT/SIT we may find ourselves able to do just that.

Chapter Eight

Dialectical Behavior Therapy and Chronic Somatization

A variant of CBT is Dialectical Behavior Therapy (DBT) developed by Marsha M. Linehan, PhD, for the management of Borderline Personality Disorder (BPD).[1] DBT has received serious attention in the professional literature for treatment of suicidal and parasuicidal (cutting, burning, and other self-abusive behaviors) individuals as well as, for instance, Binge-eating Disorder and substance abuse.[2] The current authors are also familiar with at least one hospital-based program that incorporates DBT skills training in its group psychoeducation of general psychiatric patients.[3] Although a PubMed search reveals no published data about the use of DBT in the treatment of somatization or somatoform disorders and the current authors are unaware of any studies in progress, for several reasons we find the approach intriguing and believe it warrants serious consideration for use with chronic somatization. First, personality disorders, including BPD, are frequently diagnosed in association with somatoform disorders.[4] Second, even in those cases where an Axis II diagnosis cannot be made, there are developmental factors involved in somatization which seem to mirror those which Linehan identifies with BPD.[5] Third, we believe the skills training employed in DBT targets ego deficits in the chronic somatizer which render DBT a very viable treatment option for this population. Because Linehan's description of DBT focuses on the borderline individual, our discussion will retain her terminology.

OVERVIEW OF DBT

To begin with, Linehan utilizes a biosocial model which stresses the interaction of biological and social learning influences on the development of the condition. While the precise mechanisms of emotion dysregulation in BPD are not entirely clear, Linehan states that "difficulties in limbic system reactivity and attention control may be important" factors in the etiology of the disorder.[6] Environmental factors also figure largely in the development of BPD and Linehan concentrates on the effects of what she calls the "invalidating environment." Invalidating environments are those in which an individual's private experiences are met with erratic, inappropriate, and extreme reponses.[7] Rather than confirming the appropriateness of the child's perceptions of experience, an invalidating environment may punish or trivialize them. Individuals grow up with the sense that their perceptions of reality are inaccurate or reflect socially unacceptable personality traits.[8] For example, when a child experiences distress, rather than confirm the child's perceptions as meaningful representations of experience, the environment implies they are unreliable or result from being a "bad girl" or a "bad boy." As a result, children neither learn to trust nor label their emotions and other private experiences in a way that is normative for the larger community for the same or similar experiences.[9] Since the problems of the emotionally vulnerable child are not recognized as significant, little effort is devoted to problem solving.[10] Furthermore, by "oversimplifying the ease of solving life's problems, the environment does not teach the child to tolerate distress or to form realistic goals and expectations."[11] Ironically, in the context of an invalidating environment, children often learn that it takes an extreme emotional display or an extreme problem to elicit a helpful response from parental figures.[12] We often observe the residual effects of this kind of learning in adult patients who declare that it is only by suicidal or parasuicidal behavior can they "get anyone to listen to me."

The interplay of biosocial factors results in patterns of emotional, interpersonal, and behavioral dysregulation that characterize borderline patients.[13] Emotional dysregulation refers to the tendency of borderline individuals to be highly emotionally reactive and experience depression, anxiety, irritability, and have problems with anger and its expression.[14] Interpersonal dysregulation refers to the chaotic, intense relationships and fears of abandonment often experienced by these individuals.[15] Behavioral dysregulation describes the impulsive, often self-abusive, and suicidal behaviors which characterize borderline individuals.[16] The corrective provided by DBT is a program of skills training coupled with individual psychotherapy concentrating on the areas of mindfulness, emotion regulation, interpersonal effectiveness, and distress tolerance. Skills training focuses on learning and practicing useable skills which apply specifically to one of the four targeted instructional areas. Individual therapy is structured and serves to reinforce skills application. In addition, specific problems such as suicidality are addressed in individual therapy rather than in the course of skills group. Prearranged telephone calls for therapist coaching on skills application in difficult situations is encouraged. DBT is a manualized therapy and therapists undergo training to be certified in its delivery.

DBT stresses two core strategies: Validation and problem solving. Validation is intended to communicate the message to patients that their behavior makes sense and is understandable in their present real-life situation.[17] When engaged in problem solving, the therapist engages the patient in an analysis of her behavior, enlists her in a commitment to change, and taking active steps to bring about changes in behavior.[18] The assumptions DBT makes about patients draw attention to the key role played by validation:

1. Patients are doing the best they can.
2. Patients want to improve.
3. Patients must learn new behaviors in all relevant contexts.
4. Patients cannot fail in DBT.
5. Patients may not have caused all of their own problems, but they have to solve them anyway.
6. Patients need to do better, try harder, and/or be more motivated to change.
7. The lives of suicidal, BPD individuals are unbearable as they are currently being lived.[19]

Essentially, these assumptions give the DBT patient the benefit of the doubt; rather than create an oppositional atmosphere by initially challenging a patient's behavior as problematic or pathologic, DBT validates a patient's efforts at self-regulation. Even therapy interfering behaviors such as missed appointments, unfinished homework, failure to take advantage of coaching phone calls, and the like are understood as expressing something meaningful about the patient, their coping style, and/or the therapy itself. Obviously, validation does not mean approval; validation simply recognizes that, having been raised in an invalidating environment, one's coping skills are limited and any effort to manage life stressors represents the patient's best efforts at the time; if they possessed more effective problem solving skills, they would use them. The overall effect is intended to create a collaborative relationship with the patient that facilitates healthy self-acceptance and behavioral change.

As a behavioral therapy, DBT makes use of the principles associated with operant conditioning in which learning is associated with the consequences of behavior. For example, a patient's suicidal threat elicits concern on the part of the therapist; the patient learns that empathy and concern are consequent upon threats of self-harm. This is a simple example, but it makes the point.

Other principles of operant conditioning utilized in DBT include reinforcement, punishment, and extinction. Reinforcement is a consequence that generally results in an increase of the frequency of a behavior in a given situation.[20] Reinforcement may be positive or negative. Positive reinforcement increases the likelihood of a behavior by providing positive consequences; the example of therapist-induced concern represents positive reinforcement.[21] Negative reinforcement increases the likelihood of a behavior by removing or stopping a negative or aversive stimulus.[22] The likelihood of remaining in bed in the morning is increased by pressing the snooze button on the alarm clock. Family pressures that are alleviated by illness complaints increase the probability that one will persist in the patient role.

Punishment is a consequence that results in the decrease of a behavior in a given situation and may also be positive or negative. Positive punishment functions by providing an aversive consequence to a behavior; negative punishment removes or halts a positive stimulus.[23] The use of disulfiram to trigger illness symptoms in response to alcohol consumption is a form of positive punishment, while elimination of social approval for intoxication exemplifies a negative one. Extinction is the reduction of a behavior because reinforcement is no longer provided in a given situation.[24] Once the reinforcement is withdrawn, however, an extinction burst typically occurs, marking a temporary increase in the behavior in an attempt to restore the former state of affairs. A patient's illness complaints fail to elicit the clinician's concern (withdrawal of support to promote extinction of illness-related behavior), resulting in an increase in intensity or frequency of requests for appointments, refills, and so on.

Shaping refers to the process of reinforcing successive approximations of the desired behavior.[25] Providing encouragement and praise for self-management of illness symptoms, even when tentative, is an example of shaping. By means of therapy-reinforced skills training and application and careful application of punishment, extinction of self-harmful and/or illness-related behaviors is promoted, and shaping of more effective coping behaviors takes place. Generalization refers to the application of skills outside the training session. DBT does not assume generalization will take place without difficulty and encourages use of generalization strategies to promote the process. Telephone consults, providing tapes of therapy sessions, and behavioral rehearsals are examples of generalization strategies.[26]

DBT skills training focuses on four key areas: mindfulness, emotion regulation, interpersonal effectiveness, and distress tolerance. However, before taking a look at each of these it is important to examine the behavioral analysis; that is, the Chain Analysis of Behavior, which forms the core around which the other skill areas are developed. The behavioral analysis is the central doctrine of DBT and provides insight into the context and multilevel responses which constitute the motivation for using low-level coping mechanisms. The Chain Analysis allows the patient to see how their responses to environmental stimuli often result in their use of problematic or dysfunctional coping behaviors.

By tracing the connections between a patient's individual vulnerabilities and stressful events, therapist and patient work together to help the patient understand how their response is composed of physiological, emotional, and cognitive elements which lead to the use of problem behaviors as coping devices. Evaluating the aftereffects of this behavior, patients learn how dysfunctional coping skills are self-perpetuating. Working through a behavioral analysis, whenever a patient reports having used a problem behavior, the patient learns how to employ the Chain Analysis independently and develop a greater sense of empowerment and personal responsibility.

Vulnerabilities are those conditions that render a patient likely to rely on self-harm, illness complaints, and so forth to cope with life stressors and include physical limitations, occupational stressors, and so on. The event refers to either an internal signal such as a feeling, thought, pain, and the like, or an external stressor, for instance, being informed of job loss or relationship dissolution. The physiologic response is constituted by feelings which the patient experiences in relationship to the event including changes in respiration, blood pressure, body temperature, and so forth. Cognitive responses may include cognitive distortions (black and white thinking, disastorizing, etc.), the activation of core beliefs, or memories of previous similar experiences. The emotional element describes the overall feeling response to the stressor as well as the patient's physiological state and whatever cognitive interpretations have been introduced.

Problem behaviors are coping skills which, although probably functional at one time, now cause more distress than they resolve. Aftereffects are the consequences of using the problem behavior and may be reinforcing or punishing. The combination of alcohol consumption with ingestion of analgesics may initially reduce pain awareness, but also result in hospitalization. Ultimately, the use of the behavioral analysis is solution analysis.[27] We want the patient to see how the use of DBT skills at select points along the Chain may reduce the possibility of resorting to problem behaviors. If the patient lacks the skills, the task is skills training; if the patient has the skill in their repertoire, then coaching is indicated; if the problem lies in a patient's ways of thinking, then one introduces cognitive restructuring.

Let's return to the specific DBT skill areas. Mindfulness skills derive largely from Linehan's study of Zen meditation and are intended to teach patients to observe and describe what is taking place while refraining from passing judgment on its goodness or badness.[28] Mindfulness encourages acceptance of reality in the here and now, and letting go of attachments to forcing reality to be one thing or another.[29] An example of mindfulness skills is learning to monitor one's breathing while letting go of extraneous thoughts and impressions. Employing mindfulness when a triggering event has occurred enables the patient to increase their body awareness, for example, noting where muscle tension is present, or whether they are perspiring. Mindfulness thus used as a problem-solving skill aids the patient in distancing themselves from the event so as to reduce their propensity for introducing cognitive distortions into the mix and producing extreme emotional states.

Distress tolerance skills are critical for enabling patients to learn to survive the present moment. Essentially, this means that every moment is bearable, otherwise one could not survive the unbearable moment. Distress tolerance skills enable patients to survive and tolerate crises and accept life as it is right now.[30] Specific skills include distraction techniques (exercise, reading, alternate intense sensations, social activities, etc.), self-soothing (prayer, relaxation, positive self-talk, taking a time out, etc.), and considering the pros and cons of the situation.[31] Monitoring one's breathing, the half-smile (an acceptance of reality skill), and radical acceptance (actively choosing to tolerate the moment), and willingness versus willfulness round out distress tolerance skills.[32] Some patients argue that using these skills implies approval of the situation when, in fact, they are wondering, "Shouldn't we try to change things?" Some situations are beyond immediate control, however, and willingness to accept what is and its associated distress may reduce emotional pain whereas willfulness (striving to master, control, dominate) can increase only anxiety and frustration. It's rather like beating your head against a wall; the wall isn't going to move anyway and you only end up with a headache.

Emotional lability is a well-known characteristic of many borderline patients. Indeed, from the perspective of patients, painful emotions are one of their most pressing issues. Raised in invalidating environments, these individuals are told that changing their attitude will change their emotions; that is, their emotional states result from unacceptable personality traits or having a "bad attitude."[33] To complicate the picture, the individuals sending this message often appear to have their emotions under complete, cognitive control, further frustrating the child.[34] Many of the distressing coping strategies exhibited by patients are actual attempts to manage emotional states.

> Suicidal behaviors and other dysfunctional behaviors, including substance abuse, are often behavioral solutions to intolerable painful emotions . . . In my experience, most borderline individuals try to regulate affect by simply giving themselves instructions not to feel whatever it is that they feel. This tendency is a direct result of the emotional invalidating environment, which mandates that people should smile when they are unhappy, be nice and not rock the boat when they are angry, and confess and feel forgiven when they are feeling guilty.[35]

Not infrequently, much of the borderline patient's distress comes from secondary, rather than primary, emotions.[36] Primary emotions or, in Nathanson's terms, primary affects, are often adaptive and appropriate emotional signals about the nature of experience.[37] As we discussed in chapter 5, emotion functions as a kind of psychic screening tool, enabling us to selectively focus attention. The shame, anxiety, or guilt, for example, that one feels in response to a primary emotion can be a source of considerable distress. Learning to pay mindful attention to one's emotional responses can be regarded as an exposure technique, teaching patients to tolerate their feelings without passing judgment upon them.[38]

The skills for emotion regulation include learning to identify and label emotions, identifying obstacles to changing emotions, reducing vulnerability to "emotion mind," increasing positive or pleasant emotional events, increasing mindfulness to one's current emotion, taking opposite action, and using distress tolerance techniques. Identifying and labeling emotions is critical since invalidating environments create confusion about what exactly constitutes emotional experience. The skill used here is the "emotion diary" that serves to enable patients to expand their vocabulary for a given emotion, what it feels like to have the emotion, what thoughts are often associated with it, how persons typically behave under its influence, and what are some of its aftereffects. Identifying obstacles to changing emotions helps patients identify the functions and reinforcers of an emotion.[39]

Reducing vulnerability to "emotion mind" is a technique which helps patients understand how failure to attend to physical and psychological needs—diet, sleep, illness, and the like—can increase emotional reactivity.[40] Increasing positive or pleasant emotional events is just that: Rather than allowing oneself to react randomly to whatever environmental stimuli is present, individuals should take action to provide themselves with events which trigger pleasant emotions. Increasing mindfulness to current emotion means using mindfulness to experience one's feelings without passing judgment upon them. The "basic idea here is that exposure to painful or distressing emotions, without association to negative consequences, will extinguish their ability to stimulate secondary negative emotions."[41] Taking opposite action is based on the DBT principle that emotions occur in response to stimuli. If one is experiencing a painful emotion triggered by a distressing event or sensation, the trick to reversing one's emotional state lies in providing oneself with an opposite emotional stimulus. Applying distress tolerance techniques allows patients to modulate the intensity of painful emotions, thus rendering them more manageable.[42]

Interpersonal effectiveness skills are designed to teach patients how to successfully or "effectively" manage social situations without resorting to avoidance, acting out, reliance on problem behaviors, and so forth. Specific skills include evaluating misconceptions (cognitive errors, core beliefs) about interpersonal relatedness and strategies for obtaining what one wishes without sacrificing either the relationship or one's self-respect. In some ways, interpersonal effectiveness skills are similar to assertiveness training insofar as patients learn to say "no," ask for what one needs/desires, and handle conflict. Difficulties in emotion regulation exert powerful effects on the borderline patient's interpersonal relationships.

> Borderline individuals frequently vacillate between avoidance of conflict and intense confrontation. Unfortunately, the choice of avoidance versus confrontation is based on the patient's affective state rather than on the needs of the current situation. In DBT in general, therapists challenge patient's negative expectancies regarding their environment, their relationships, and themselves. The therapists should assist the patients in learning to apply specific interpersonal problem-solving, social, and assertiveness skills to modify aversive environments and develop effective relationships.[43]

DBT skills and the problems they address are not unidimensional; just as an individual's difficulties in functioning affect multiple areas, skills with specific application to one area ultimately impact the patient in others as well.

DBT differs from traditional CBT in several ways. To begin with, DBT stresses acceptance of behavior and reality as it is.[44]

> To a great extent . . . standard cognitive-behavioral therapy can be thought of as a technology of change. It derives many of its techniques from the field of learning, which is the study of behavioral change through experience. In contrast, DBT emphasizes the importance of balancing change with acceptance. Although acceptance of patients as they are is crucial to any good therapy DBT goes a step further than the standard cognitive-behavioral therapy in emphasizing the necessity of teaching patients to accept themselves and their world as it is in the moment. Thus, a technology of acceptance is as important as the technology of change.[45]

Second, the attention paid in DBT to therapy-interfering behaviors such as self-abuse is more akin to the psychodynamic concept of transference than it is to any emphasis common to CBT.[46] Analysis of patient behaviors which interrupt or otherwise interfere with the process of therapy are examples of material which is addressed in individual DBT psychotherapy. A third difference which Linehan stresses is her emphasis on the therapeutic relationship as critical to progress in DBT. This emphasis is echoed in the assumptions DBT makes about therapy:

1. The most caring thing a therapist can do is help patients change in ways that bring them closer to their own ultimate goals.
2. Clarity, precision, and compassion are of the utmost importance in the conduct of DBT.
3. The therapeutic relationship is a real relationship between equals.
4. Principles of behavior are universal, affecting therapists no less than patients.
5. DBT therapists can fail.
6. DBT can fail even if therapists do not.
7. Therapists treating BPD patients need support.[47]

Unlike other directive-type modalities in which the therapist often takes on the role of "teacher" and the patient as "student," and in which there is generally an unequal distribution of power, Linehan insists that DBT therapy not perpetuate the power differential that often characterizes most of the borderline patient's other relationships.[48] Because of the residual effects of being raised in an invalidating environment, borderline patients may respond to the inherent inequalities in therapy by exhibiting overly dependent or overly independent behaviors.[49] Admittedly, any psychotherapy involves some measure of inequality. For example, while therapy is often a very intimate experience in terms of patient disclosure, there are limits on the kind and degree of therapist self-disclosure. One pays for therapy; it is a professional relationship. However, it an effort to navigate even the basic inequalities present in therapy, borderline patients may oscillate between excessive neediness and appearing to reject the therapist. By maintaining a here and now relationship as between relative equals and respecting the patient's power within therapy, DBT offers a corrective to the patient's behavioral extremes and permits therapy to act as a model of healthy interpersonal relatedness. Linehan notes that, while CBT therapists certainly affirm the importance of a collaborative relationship between therapist and patient, in her experience with suicidal patients, the therapeutic relationship itself is often the most important element that ensures patient safety.[50]

Finally, DBT is distinguished from traditional CBT by its emphasis on dialectics.[51] The dialectical approach of thesis-antithesis-synthesis was developed by the nineteenth-century German philosopher G. W. F. Hegel and found its more commonly known application in the Dialectical Materialism of Karl Marx and Friedrich Engels.[52] While behavior therapy also stresses process over structure, DBT takes this concept much further. The therapeutic relationship nurtured by DBT is, in its essence, dialectical.

> From the point of view of dialogue and relationship, "dialectics" refers to change by persuasion and by making use of the oppositions inherent in the therapeutic

> relationship, rather than by formal impersonal logic. Thus, unlike analytical thinking, dialectics is personal, taking into account and affecting the total person. It is an approach to engaging a person in dialogue so that movement can be made. Through the therapeutic relationship of contradictory positions, both patient and therapist can arrive at new meanings within old meaning.[53]

Following a dialectical perspective, as change is fostered in the patient, both therapy and therapist are transformed.

DBT AND CHRONIC SOMATIZATION

The biosocial model is a useful one for thinking about somatization. Certainly a number of biological processes are involved in its development including the endocrine and immune systems, amino acids, and neurotransmitters. Perception and the communication of body signals no doubt figure into the picture. But experimental investigations dealing with the interaction of behavioral changes, biological variations, and body perceptions are rare, reflecting the need for further exploration into the neurophysiology of somatization.[54] Thus, apart from what do we know about functional somatic syndromes, our knowledge about the neurophysiology of somatization is still in the inferential stages and, for now, that will have to do.

Although the term "invalidating environment" is generally absent in the literature on somatization, Stuart and Noyes make an interesting argument for the contribution of developmental factors in the etiology of somatoform disorders. They hypothesize that anxious attachment with caregivers during childhood and early exposure to illness increase the likelihood that distress will be manifested somatically.[55] As noted above, children raised in invalidating environments learn that ordinary problems are insufficient to elicit concern from parents and other careproviders. Instead, it takes an extreme display of emotion or distress to communicate one's need for assistance. If emotional concerns are minimized or otherwise invalidated in childhood and illness is validated as an appropriate cause for parental care, it is not unreasonable to postulate individuals will retain this behavior into adulthood. Stuart and Noyes also note that if somatizers' interpersonal interactions with others, including physicians, ultimately lead to rejection, this reinforces the somatizer's belief that he or she will be abandoned.[56] Fears of abandonment leading to frequent, intense relationships has long been considered a diagnostic criterion for BPD. In the case of an individual which has formed anxious attachment with careproviders, the expectation that their needs will provoke rejection may provoke automatic thoughts about the physician, for instance, "He doesn't believe me, he's going to refuse to help me, etc." This type of thinking may precipitate early discontinuation of treatment, medical noncompliance, and doctor shopping. The guardedness which we often observe in somatizing patients may very well reflect early experiences with careproviders in what we suggest may be considered an invalidating environment. This is not to say every somatizing patient has experienced anxious attachment; there are a number of factors implicated in the development of somatization. Nevertheless, environmental and developmental considerations warrant serious attention.

The core strategies of validation and problem solving are of particular interest in the treatment of somatization. As we've noted previously, the tendency for the doctor-patient relationship to become adversarial is common when dealing with somatizers and the idea of validating a patient's perceptions and efforts at coping may seem novel. Spouses and family members often report feeling frustrated while trying to deal with a somatizing relative; there is an inclination to blame the patient for failing to "try hard enough to get well." Such interpersonal interactions may be perceived by the patient as invalidating. For clinicians to openly recognize that somatizers are actually doing the best they can, given their histories and life circumstances, goes a long way to reduce tension in the examining room.

Following DBT theory, we presume patients actually do wish to improve and previous so-called treatment failures may represent an inadequate therapeutic alliance, lack of understanding of the patient's illness conceptions, impatience with progress, rather than absence of motivation. The inability of these patients to solve problems effectively results, not from stubbornness or resistance, but from a lack of skills. Raised in settings that may approximate an invalidating environment by parents who may have little in the way of problem-solving skills themselves, it is hardly surprising that somatizers seem vulnerable to life stressors. To a great extent, we may assume they simply don't know what to do. What complicates our understanding of the difficulty somatizers have with problem solving is a concept called apparent competency. Patients present a façade of functionality, but under stress, their ability to cope breaks down.[57] They may look better than they actually are and we may be misled into colluding with their insistence that they've been doing "just fine" until this or that illness derailed them. As with borderline patients, the somatizer's functionality may be variable and conditional upon circumstances.[58] Poor problem-solving and coping skills inhibits the generalization of the somatizer's competency across a variety of life situations. As with the borderline patient, this underlying inadequacy is demonstrated in areas involving interpersonal relations, emotion regulation, and distress tolerance.

Validation implies recognition that using problem behaviors to manage distress is a functional behavior. The outcome of such behavior may be damaging to self-esteem, appearance, overall health, and a host of other factors; this doesn't change the fact that the intent is related to coping. One of the typical responses patients offer when asked why they persist in a problem behavior is, "I don't know." By working through a Chain Analysis, the clinician can help the patient understand the interplay of factors which results in symptom exacerbation, desperate calls to the physician, social withdrawal, and the like. Since somatizers are so exquisitely sensitive to bodily sensations, information about emotions and cognitions is especially useful here. Often these individuals are unaware of the thoughts that accompany their response to stress. Techniques of CBT can be quite helpful in isolating automatic thoughts, gathering information to test their validity, suggesting alternative interpretations, and so forth. Because alexithymia is so evident in somatizing patients, identification of emotions and their place in the stress response may be rather alien to the somatizer. Invalidating environments not only provoke extreme emotional expressions, they also promote repression of emotion in some individuals. Fear of being taken over by emotion and losing control, becoming unacceptable, and being rejected inhibit emotional awareness. The Chain Analysis provides an opportunity for normalizing experience and placing physical sensation, emotion, and cognition into a larger context, effectively introducing the patient to a practical awareness of the mind-body interface.

The application of DBT skills training begins with mindfulness. Somatizing patients often balk at the notion that "meditation" can help manage physical discomfort, and the clinician does well to address this objection from the outset. It is important to stress that mindfulness is about developing a mindset of acceptance. Explaining how techniques such as monitoring one's breathing or concentrating on a pleasant physical sensation (holding a piece of candy in one's mouth and observing how it melts slowly, what are the flavors, etc.) are intended to instruct patients in focusing their attention can be helpful. Acceptance is difficult for somatizing patients because they are accustomed to thinking about their symptoms in judgmental terms and labeling them as indicative of severe illness—hence, symptoms are "bad" and should be eliminated. Learning to accept the presence of pain or distress and withholding judgment ultimately has the effect of enabling a patient to develop a greater sense of tolerance. While we generally don't refer to mindfulness as a distress tolerance technique, it can function this way by teaching patients to "be with" their symptoms and refrain from cognitive distortions like catastrophizing. By focusing on developing a "wise mind" that incorporates awareness of cognition and emotion, patients also learn to avoid intellectualizing their discomfort or falling into "emotion mind" which may lead to extreme emotional expressions and heightened illness-related anxiety. Wise mind adds the element of intuition to emotional experiencing and logical analysis. Linehan's comments are instructive in this regard:

> In effect, (patients) have to let go of emotional processing and logical analysis, of set ideas and extreme reactions; they must become calm enough to allow wise knowing to proceed uncomplicated and unintruded on by other, more volitional ("reasonable mind") or overdetermined ("emotion mind") modes of knowing.[59]

Nurturing a wise-minded approach to illness helps patients feel more empowered and less vulnerable to what they perceive to be the whims of their condition.

Distress tolerance skills are met with a mixed reaction by many patients. Some embrace the idea of utilizing distraction or self-soothing to take their minds off their pain. Others tend to scoff at the idea that "reading a book" or "taking a hot bath" can make a difference; their suffering is too severe, too "medical" to rely on "pop psych" for relief. We might expect dependent or overlyconventional types to represent the first response, hypernormals and autocratic-managerials the second. This makes a great deal of sense: We expect dependent and overlyconventional types to wish to follow the therapist's lead and appear obliging and pleasant. Hypernormal and autocratic types experience strong power drives and expressing opposition enables them to distance themselves from feelings of vulnerability. The power drive shows up for many hypernormal and autocratic types in their insistence that their condition is "too serious" to respond to the kinds of techniques that might help someone with a lesser condition. There is almost a narcissistic element involved here that suggests, "I am too special, important, powerful, to have an ordinary illness." In any case, comments such as these can't be dismissed; validation of the patient's experience dictates that we understand they are doing the best they can under the circumstances. Leading these patients through a distraction technique such as holding a piece of ice very tightly in one's hand for as long as possible demonstrates the power of an alternate physical sensation to reduce distress over one's discomfort. Asking patients to select specific distraction or self-soothing skills which they affirm they will use at home, and then assigning homework to use the skills and record their observations, can also serve to enlist the patient as a partner in a personal empirical study. Evaluating their successes and failures in the next class meeting creates a feeling of camaraderie, a sense that patient and therapist are working collaboratively to arrive at workable skills to increase tolerance of distressing sensations and stressful circumstances.

Emotion regulation skills focus on developing awareness of and comfort with affective states. In ways similar to borderline patients, we observe that somatizers have difficulty identifying and labeling emotions. As stated in chapter 7, alexithymia tends to be a characteristic of many somatizing patients and is well addressed by emotion regulation skills. For some individuals the lack of emotional awareness seems to focus attention on physical sensation as a source of knowledge about internal states. Anger, fear, sadness, and other negative emotions may be thus misinterpreted as pain or physical distress. Learning how to correctly identify and tolerate one's affective state can be a real boon for the somatizer. In addition, since alexithymia may promote acting out behaviors, learning emotion regulation skills can enable more functional expression of needs, desires, discomfort, and so forth. Patients with hypernormal personality traits may have considerable difficulty expressing painful emotions when perceived as reflecting antisocial tendencies or attitudes. Anger, fear, and shame may be denied or projected onto family or careproviders, generating stress and anxiety. As a result, the patient may imagine herself as misunderstood or socially unacceptable, activating fears of abandonment. Learning how to accurately identify one's emotions and assume responsibility for their regulation can reduce interpersonal stress, defensiveness, and reliance on physical symptoms to enable avoidance of social contact.

Interpersonal effectiveness skills target the somatizing patient's characteristic tendency to either avoid interpersonal situations or handle them poorly. Both behaviors involve misconceptions about the meaning of interpersonal communication. Addressing these misconceptions is the first step in interpersonal effectiveness skill training. By allowing patients to identify their personal attitudes about relating to others, we offer them the opportunity to experience validation from both the clinician and the skills group as well as help them rephrase their misconceptions in ways that are more empowering. Skills that follow include learning how to grade one's responses to a request and communicate assertively while maintaining a relationship and one's self-respect. Raised in apparently invalidating environments, one learns to say "yes" or "no" without qualification and without regard to one's own preferences. Grading responses teaches patients to consider their own needs and feelings about a situation. They learn to evaluate interpersonal encounters using criteria such as timeliness, capability, and appropriateness to a relationship. Such a process reduces uncertainty and helps generate a sense of competency. Assertive communication training provides patients with a structured interview approach for addressing other persons. Elements such as stating the facts, expressing your emotions about the situation, asking for what you wish/saying no to another's request, reinforcing the consequences of having your position respected, and negotiating are included in this skill. As with the other skill areas, homework assignments are provided for practice and personal evaluation.

While skills training classes incorporate role-playing and skills practice opportunities, individual therapy and telephone consultations are often the best way for individual skills application. During a weekly session, for example, the therapist will approach a patient's difficulty communicating with her physician by asking how she might use a particular DBT skill to make her point. The same process might take place in a telephone conversation, this time prior to meeting with the physician, in order to plan in advance for a more optimal outcome. It is important, not only for therapists to be thoroughly familiar with somatization, but to also undergo training in DBT if they are going to see somatizers who are participating in DBT skills training. Familiarity with the theory is helpful, but also one needs to know how to coach skills application and this implies thorough familiarity with the entire approach.

Skills training and individual DBT therapy are, essentially, modes of developing ego strength. We have discussed how chronic somatization is a disorder affecting ego functioning in which illness operates as an ego-integrating factor. While we do not expect DBT to resolve somatization, we do believe development in each of the DBT skill areas serves as a corrective to ego deficits. We rightly conceive the healthy ego as the psychic agent enabling effective management of interpersonal stresses, regulating affective states, and promoting toleration of distressing circumstances. If we understand somatization of the chronic type as a disorder resulting from an interaction of biological and environmental factors resulting in ego deficits which inhibit affective processing, distress tolerance, and interpersonal relatedness, then DBT has the potential to be of considerable help to the somatizing patient.

PRACTICAL TREATMENT CONSIDERATIONS

Setting up a DBT program for the treatment of somatization requires, above all, a ready patient population base. Experience has taught the current writers that this population tends to have a fairly high drop-out rate and for a group to be viable, there must be patients "waiting in the wings," so to speak. For this reason, we believe an academic medical center is, perhaps, the most ideal setting for a group of this type. Teaching hospitals tend to see a large number of high-acuity patients and those with somatoform disorders or functional somatic syndromes are not uncommon. Academic centers are ideal locations for instruction in the diagnosis and management of somatization. In addition, staffing considerations are fairly easily addressed. Residents-in-training are actively involved in following patients and provide ready pharmacological assistance. Social workers, psychologists, and other allied mental health personnel can undergo DBT training, lead groups, and provide individual psychotherapy. Patients often feel closely tied to providers in these settings and being enlisted in a DBT group may seem more like a natural extension of their regular care. Non-academic medical centers and community mental health clinics are not excluded from starting DBT programs for somatoform disorders. The ability to do so, however, depends once again on an available patient population base. In our experience, non-academic hospitals and mental health centers depend on the physician community for referrals and, while these are often good referral sources, patients very often fail to arrive for an initial intake. Unless a program has a large number of referrals, it will never progress beyond the drawing table.

The next question is pragmatic: How does one decide which patients to assign to DBT? Several factors will influence a clinician's decision in this regard. While a DBT program would certainly be helpful for a patient that is uncomfortable in group settings, this patient might benefit most from at least a short course of individual CBT/CBMT therapy. Once completed, if the patient wishes additional practical training, referral to a DBT group could be appropriate. Time is another factor: DBT groups generally meet for twenty-six weeks (two hours/week skills training) with an hour of individual therapy per week. Some patients may be unwilling or unable to make such a commitment because of child care or other considerations.

Limitations on insurance coverage may necessitate some patients seek individual therapy even if they wish to enter a DBT group. If a patient has a limited number of outpatient mental health visits available in a calendar year, there may be inadequate coverage to pay for DBT, rendering individual therapy the obvious choice. Parity clauses, of course, extend coverage since parity mental health diagnoses (e.g., Major Depression, Bipolar Disorder, Schizophrenia, Obsessive-Compulsive Disorder) are considered major medical conditions. Parity clauses, however, are not uniform in managed care; not every policy is required to offer a parity clause. While it can be argued that somatization is a quasi-medical condition, that is, a medical condition with psychiatric elements, the problem of obtaining authorization for treatment remains. An alternative involves the diagnosis of depression or an anxiety disorder secondary to a general medical condition. While these are not generally considered parity diagnoses, such an approach stresses that treatment is directed at the attending psychiatric symptoms rather than the underlying somatization. If depression is recurrent or meets criteria for Major Depressive Disorder or Generalized Anxiety Disorder, then a parity clause is activated.

Discussions with managed care providers leads the current authors to believe there is genuine interest in providing treatment for somatizing patients. The cost of maintaining these patients on a treatment-as-usual basis can be exorbitant, but treatment programs are a new concept and, frankly, insurance carriers are just as uncertain as clinicians as to how billing and payment should be managed. The patient, unfortunately, is caught in the middle of this dilemma and the decision to refer to DBT or individual therapy often hinges on what kind of insurance provisions the patient has available.

A fourth consideration relates to comorbidity. Obviously, patients with comorbid personality disorders, especially BPD, are good candidates for DBT. As long as a patient is committed to a DBT program and insurance poses no limitations, we are inclined to regard this as the treatment of choice. Furthermore, even if there is no obvious character pathology, we believe DBT offers potential for a very good therapeutic outcome for most somatizing patients.

Current modes of treatment are also important issues to evaluate. If a patient is receiving supportive therapy, for example, and has a solid alliance established with their current therapist, it does not generally make good clinical sense to refer the patient elsewhere. If the therapist has training in the delivery of CBT or CBMT, then gradually incorporating these elements in therapy with a view to symptom management would be appropriate. If the therapist is DBT certified, there is no reason why individual skills training cannot take place as well. Referral from an existing therapist would likely be indicated if, for instance, a therapeutic impasse had developed and could not be resolved or the therapist was unfamiliar with somatization and/or related syndromes and believed the patient would be better served elsewhere. Psychopharmacology is an important aspect of treating the chronic somatizer and the reader is referred to chapter 10 for a discussion of medication management.

The degree of familiarity with and commitment to treatment options on the part of the referring clinician will impact patient participation a great deal. It is assumed that a referring physician will continue to provide medical care for a patient who has been referred for psychological treatment. If the patient gains the impression that their physician does not regard therapy as important or seems only mildly interested in what the patient is learning, it will be much easier for the patient to imagine herself dissatisfied and discontinue therapy. One must remember that for most somatizing patients, their primary alliance is with the medical provider. It takes time for elements of this alliance to be transferred to a group or individual therapy. Until a patient has established a connection with the provider of psychological services, their relationship to therapy is tenuous. To ensure compliance, it is critical that physicians communicate support for the patient by showing an active interest in what they are learning and how successful they are in generalizing the material. Accordingly, referring physicians must take the time to familiarize themselves with their patients' therapy. A number of resources are available for this purpose and many offer continuing medical education units as incentives for participation.

Ironically, when these patients are referred for therapy, it is often because they've reached a stalemate with their doctor. We would argue that therapy should not be regarded as a either a last resort or corrective to patient resistance. As our osteopathic colleagues frequently remind us, effective treatment involves mind and spirit as well as body. Therapy for somatizing patients should be considered from the outset as an important element in the overall treatment plan. In the selection of a therapist there is a distinct advantage to working with non-prescribing clinicians. Some patients may regard a physician/therapist as a source of new or different medications in the hope of finding the "magic pill." By working with psychologists, social workers, and the like, one eliminates the potential for "splitting" therapist and medical doctor over the issue of medications. In the event one wishes to refer to a psychiatrist for psychoactive medications as well as therapy, the prescribing clinicians will have to work closely to minimize "splitting."

We have stressed the importance of personality theory for understanding the process of somatization. To what extent can interpersonal theory serve as an aid for evaluating patients for psychotherapy? Leary has gone to some pains to suggest how certain personality types are more or less likely to enter and/or complete psychotherapy as well as comment upon proclivities for therapy-interfering behavior. Overlyconventional patients, for example, will seem agreeable and cooperative, but their repression or denial of Level III traits results in a therapy lacking depth and positive change. With somatizing patients, however, we don't really have the luxury of screening patients for therapy based on personality considerations. We want them in treatment and the primary obstacle we face is motivation. Convincing this population that psychological treatments are in their best interest is a tough proposition and once we have secured a commitment to therapy, we don't want to sabotage our gains by demonstrating reticence about its outcome. It is more helpful to use the elements of interpersonal theory to help us target ego deficits, establish measurable goals for therapy, and manage therapy-interfering behaviors. For example, with an overlyconventional personality type, we want to address dysfunctional core beliefs about assertiveness and the value of experiencing/expressing painful emotions. Dependent types generally reveal narcissistic traits at Level III; in group situations, these traits may show up as criticism of other patients and are then followed by missed appointments and withdrawal from therapy. Mindful that the dependent's narcissism is defensive in nature and serves to reduce anxiety about taking responsibility for independent functioning, the clinician highlights the advantages of being in a group where support and assistance with problem solving are available. The hypernormal type may dismiss therapy, particularly group therapy, after only a few sessions on the grounds that the other members have "mental problems" and the hypernormal, of course, does not. By validating the patient's concerns and stressing the functional nature of DBT skills training and so forth, the clinician focuses on the behavioral aspects of therapy. The hypernormal needs to understand that therapy is designed to help them cope with their symptoms in a more, rather than less, functional manner. Essentially, we appeal to their sense of duty and responsibility to enable them to embrace therapy as the "right thing to do" for themselves and their families. From the standpoint of treatment, interpersonal theory is highly pragmatic; it provides us with a means of supporting treatment compliance that can be easily missed by over-reliance on other theoretical persuasions.

Symptom becomes disease when illness becomes a way of life. In the case of the chronic-type of somatizing patient, illness provides an ego-integrating factor that is highly resistant to change. We have discussed CBT, CBMT, and DBT as symptom management therapies intended to reduce such problem behaviors as frequent and urgent calls to the physician, abuse of analgesic medications, social avoidance, and the like, and promote greater individual capability and responsibility. At Level II, patients want to experience the resolution and elimination of illness; at Level III, however, they desperately cling to their symptoms to maintain some degree of functionality. The goal of behavioral therapies is not the removal of somatization, but the development of skills which reduce the patient's reliance upon somatization and promote a more meaningful lifestyle.

Chapter Nine

The Situational Somatizing Patient in Treatment

Pragmatically speaking, our ultimate concern for thinking about somatization is to determine the most meaningful treatment options. For the situational somatizer, these are typically far more promising, as well as intriguing, than those for the chronic type. As the reader may imagine, the reason for this lies in the fact that, while situational somatizers may indeed experience some long-term deleterious effects of somatization, in general, it does not serve to provide personality organization like it does for the chronic patient. When used as a defensive strategy against the anxiety associated with the eruption of Level III traits into conscious experience, somatization is less virulent than it is when relied upon as a primary means of coping with life stressors. In our experience, situational somatizers are anxious, worried, and frightened persons who are desperately trying to maintain their self-identity as functional individuals. As we have pointed out, chronic somatizers seem to stubbornly cling to somatization as a kind of buffer between themselves and life. In a sense, the chronic somatizer is able to function because of somatization; that is, it is a way of bolstering the patient's fragile ego so that s/he can function at a level that matches his or her overall capabilities. Should it be any wonder that somatization of the chronic type is a daunting adversary? This is not to say the situational somatizer is easy to treat; far from it. However, what concerns us is not ease of treatment, but response to treatment, and we are more optimistic about the potential outcomes for this subtype. As stated earlier in this volume, situational somatization represents a response to life events which carry the weight of an existential crisis. The treatment of choice for situational somatization is short-term existential psychotherapy. However, before we discuss the details of this approach, we think it will be helpful for the reader if we explain how we arrived at this conclusion and offer a brief introduction to existential thinking.

FOLLOWING THE PATIENT

In our search for an appropriate treatment for situational somatization, we determined from the outset to follow the "road less traveled," so to speak, instead of our own particular therapeutic preferences. Thus, we hoped to avoid what we believe has been a procedural error in the development of less-effective therapies. Rather than adopt a treatment with which we were most familiar and try to adapt patients to match our approach, we have looked to our patients and their pathology and allowed these to guide our work. In this way, we have followed the lead of Edmund Husserl (1859–1938), who questioned the Cartesian dichotomy of mind and body which splits reality into subject and object that we discussed in chapter 3. Instead, Husserl argued that we need to understand the world "as it is experienced in our consciousness, as distinct from viewing it as being constituted of remote entities that are in some way separate to our perception of them."[1] He used the concept of "bracketing," to describe how we can insulate an object of inquiry from our predispositions and allow it to be itself.[2]

Freud was similarly convinced that the analyst should avoid attempting to influence the patient's psychological processes of the patient. For this reason, he insisted the analyst sit behind the patient, who reclined on a couch and spoke whatever came to mind (free association), freed from interference by the analyst's facial expressions, and so forth. In actuality, the notion of "complete analytic objectivity" is actually more fiction than fact because the mere presence of the analyst constitutes an alteration of the patient's experience. Since our presence in the examination room exerts some influence on patients, we resist approaching them and their illness complaints as though they were simply objects of inquiry. In so doing, we avoid creating a reductive and dehumanizing effect that may reinforce the patient's belief that their symptoms are distinct from their overall experience of themselves as human beings. We bracket our Cartesian categories and ways of thinking and permit ourselves to enter into the distress, misery, fearfulness, and bewilderment motivating the patient's desire for relief. We forge a relationship built upon receptivity and trust—not only the patient's trust in us, but also our trust in them to lead us appropriately through the process of discovery and treatment.

Accordingly, throughout this volume we have resisted the notion that somatization in all its forms can be regarded as something that could be treated in isolation from the patient's experience. Instead, we have tried to understand why individuals somatize in the first place. It is paradoxical that a patient who valued their functional life would seek to prolong disease recovery with somatizing symptoms. One would actually expect these patients to be eager to experience a rapid recovery, yet this is not the case. What is it about surgery that creates such anxiety or dread that some patients experience an ongoing distress or debilitation that has no clear etiology in the treatment itself? Are we dealing with a lack of knowledge on the part of the patient? Clearly, if knowledge was the problem, then somatization could be resolved simply by thorough explanations by the clinician. Even the most competent and careful physicians, however, have patients who become somatizers. Something else is at work and we are convinced it relates to the patient's unconscious perceptions about the meaning of the medical procedure and its effect on their personality structure and mode of functioning in the world.

INTRODUCTION TO EXISTENTIAL THINKING

Normally, when there is congruency or harmony between individuals' unconscious motivations and conscious desires, resiliency is also evident in their ability to cope with life's vicissitudes. When congruency between conscious and unconscious is absent, an individual experiences an inner discord that results in a sense of self-estrangement. In layman's terms, we might say these individuals are not in touch with themselves or lack self-awareness. But it goes far deeper than this: The absence of a sense of intrapersonal integrity results in a variety of dysfunctional behaviors including interpersonal hostilities. We turn our intolerance of our own weaknesses into a bitter prejudice against persons whom we perceive to be different from ourselves. Werner Wolff describes this as a "crisis of personality, which is not a product of the time we live in, nor a product of upbringing and experience; it is a product of our very existence . . . (a) crisis in this sense puts at stake the meaning and position which man gives to his life."[3] At a deep symbolic level, such a crisis threatens not only an individual's personality organization, but also their very existence. In short, the patient experiences an existential crisis.

When we use the term "existential," we are referring to situations which challenge our normal patterns of living. We all engage in problem solving in a variety of ways. Perhaps the car has an unexpected flat tire or the baby has a cold and we must decide who will stay home to care for it. While problems such as these are inconvenient or irritating, they don't generally pose a challenge to our personal identity; we manage them and go on. Of course, we do not mean to minimize the impact of daily life upon individual coping styles nor do we wish to neglect the emotional dysregulation that characterizes the responses of individuals with personality disorders to life problems. Our point is, that as distressing as some situations may seem, there tends to be an ontological difference between the event that challenges our patience and the one which strikes at the heart of who we are as persons.

Existential problems interrupt daily life and call attention to its quality. They generate not only an uncomfortable awareness that our lives are unfulfilling but associated feelings of guilt and anxiety. Guilt feelings emerge because we sense that we have failed at various points to live up to our potential, and anxiety because we realize time is not always on our side. We may begin to question whether our lives express meaning and purpose. Ordinarily, the day-to-day routine allows us some welcome respite from questions such as these: The office, socializing with friends, our children's soccer games, as worthy as they are, may actually lull us into a false sense of security. We may even try to fill our lives with activity that acts like a drug that dulls the psychic senses and allows us to think, "I'm doing alright and life is good." The existential questions haven't vanished in the meantime; they've simply been driven into the unconscious, where they haunt our dreams and may drive us to neurotic behaviors such as addiction, workaholism, and frenetic consumerism.[4] Karl Jaspers argued that "suffering and the poignancy of our limitations are what keep us real and alive . . . awareness of these situations, together with wonder and doubt, is the beginning of our becoming ourselves . . . paradoxically, people are inclined to hide and obscure these truths to themselves—and thus drift away from self-knowledge and into pathology."[5] An existential crisis occurs when circumstances force the questions of meaning and truth into conscious awareness and we have no where to run and there is no place left to hide.

Generally we think of existential crises resulting from something perceived as life threatening such as the diagnosis of a terminal illness or the loss of a loved one. In point of fact, however, an existential crisis can have multiple etiologies because we all have our own basic existential problems to solve and we all have to come to grips with the human drive for self-completion. There is little doubt that personality plays a significant role in determining the kinds of existential issues with which we are confronted. The overlyconventional types, for example, have to confront the fact that conformity and people-pleasing may have left them without a well-defined personal identity. Hypernormal and managerial types are forced to address powerlessness and dependency. Notice that these issues are very similar to the Level III traits that these types unconsciously repress. We don't believe this is accidental; fulfillment as an individual is closely tied with wholeness, and wholeness is inextricably bound with the acceptance of those aspects of our personalities which we find least acceptable.

SOMATIZATION AND EXISTENTIAL CRISIS

One of the basic tenants of existential philosophy is that human beings are essentially alone in the world.[6] We cope with existential solitude and strive for completion by establishing relationships, having children, and engaging in creative activity, the ultimate expression of which is the re-creation of ourselves. We do this by frankly addressing the questions about our presence, significance, and place in the world. Neurosis represents an unsuccessful attempt at re-creating the self because it short-circuits existential conflict. Neurosis blocks the necessary confrontation with existential questions and the need for self-acceptance and affirmation by which we live in any genuine sense. In essence, it substitutes symptoms for awareness and once these are present, the patient's focus shifts from fear, anxiety, or guilt, to symptom relief. Patients thus prove to themselves that they are sick and need treatment. As long as the "illness" is present, there is no need to confront existential issues. There is always the danger that an individual, especially those prone to somatization, will try to circumvent the existential crisis by resorting to a neurotic solution. The result may be a life dominated by the perception of illness.

Psychological defenses come into play as responses to therapeutic goals which are perceived, not infrequently, as a source of considerable distress.[7] It is the nature of the psyche to prompt us to become whole, well-integrated, healthy-minded individuals. To help accomplish this task, the unconscious strives to become conscious. One of the telltale signs that we are treading the unknown territory of the unconscious is a sense of dread. In contrast to fear which is usually related to something specific, dread is the deep, chilling fear of nonbeing.[8] It is the fear of losing oneself and ceasing to exist. We might even go so far as to say that dread is the fear of decompensation, the loss of the conscious self in psychosis and madness. We described in chapter 6 how the hypernormal, overlyconventional, autocratic/managerial, and passive-dependent personality types take great pains to defend themselves against progressive disorganization or the unconscious fear of decompensation and loss of functioning. For these personalities, the inability to function normally is tantamount to ceasing to exist in any meaningful way. And meeting the unconscious aspects of the self carries with it the fear of being overwhelmed, of being swept away by a tidal wave of uncontrollable affect. When we feel overwhelmed by the possibility of knowing ourselves as we truly are, our defenses intervene to "save us."

The mind's own therapeutic goal is to motivate us to integrate those aspects of ourselves which we have least interest in knowing into conscious awareness. The therapeutic function of the existential crisis is to bring us face to face with these unacceptable aspects of our personalities. It is possible, however, that our defenses may actually become a barrier between us and wholeness. We might call this the dark side of psychological defenses because, while they enable us to cope with life in some very effective ways, they can also cause us to become entrenched in behaviors or ways of thinking that are decidedly dysfunctional. Of course, we're referring to neurotic solutions. For some individuals, somatization is the defense par excellence. It is for this reason, that somatization can be so ultimately damaging: It protects the ego but it cripples the personality.

EXISTENCE AND PERCEPTION

Why one person will be debilitated by illness and another is not comes down to perception and, as we pointed out in chapter 5, perception is an ego function. Appearance and existence can be two very different things. An individual may appear to be happy and well adjusted while, at the same time, covering up a miserable existence. Appearance and existence are also reflected in sensory experience. Consider, for example, the flag of the United States. In appearance, it is a construction of needle, threat, and material that presents a configuration of red and white stripes as well as white stars on a blue field. When it passes in review, however, persons place their right hands over their hearts, men remove their hats, and some will cheer. It isn't the flag itself that prompts such behavior: It is the meaning with which it is invested that leads women and men to fight and die for it. Not every person who sees the American flag attributes it with this kind of value. A citizen of another country might understand that the flag represents a sociopolitical entity but they could hardly be expected to regard it with the emotional intensity that characterizes the average American. Such is the nature and role of symbols in the human psyche.

A symbol is more than a mere representation; symbols participate in the reality for which they stand, and this is why they are so powerful.[9] Symbols indicate one's values and have the ability to evoke an affective response. We attribute or project tremendous meaning onto certain symbols and these projections have the power not only to alter our perceptions, but also to challenge our existence as well. Symbols do not determine perception; symbolic content is determined by perception. Symbols reflect our interpretations of them and we become rigid in our thinking when we cannot separate the two. Individuals who cannot—or will not—recognize, for instance, the essential difference between the American flag and their personal valuation of it may well be intolerant of those who do not share their perceptions. Intolerance is a defensive position which allows the individual to avoid confronting the ambivalence that is inherent in opposing views. We might even say that intolerance is a way of shoring up a weak ego and preventing the eruption into consciousness of intolerable affects.

Let's take this a step further. Consider, for example, a hypernormal individual who, true to type, values his capability and willingness to accept responsibility. He prides himself in the fact that he never misses a day of work and he's succeeded in putting his children through college. Although generous to a fault and supportive of his favorite charities, he would never admit to the weakness or dependency he associates with individuals requiring charity. Suddenly his world begins to fall apart when he is diagnosed with an illness requiring surgery. He has nightmares of himself in a wheelchair and his spouse standing on a street corner with a sign reading, "Will clean houses for food." While he tries to shake off his misgivings about the surgery, once it is completed he begins experiencing post-operative pain that prevents his return to work. While the physician can find no reason for the ongoing discomfort, the patient continues to complain of muscle weakness, loss of sleep, and pain that is unresponsive to medication. Our patient has identified himself with that which symbolizes his life and values; that is, his way of being in the world, his responsible character, his ability to provide for his family. In his mind, these constitute his identity, and with the possibility of even a temporary loss of function due to surgical recovery, his existential fears of debilitation have taken over. According to his perception, illness signifies dependence and dependence signifies death. The unanswered questions of the meaning of his existence begin to erode his typical defenses and, in a last-ditch effort to avoid dealing with himself, he unconsciously substitutes a symptom for genuine awareness. His ego integrity remains intact, his Level III contents (dependence, etc.) remain buried in the unconscious, and he turns to his physician for assistance.

Like the individual who cannot separate symbol from perception, somatizing patients cannot separate illness from perception. The maintenance of the perception of illness is essential to prevent a breakdown of existential proportions. It really does come down to perception. The existence of an event "is not necessarily defined by it's appearance or by its elements but by the interrelationship of the elements and the perception of existence is not necessarily defined by the sensory, palpable, and conscious processes of the observer but rather by the interrelationships of these and other processes in the observer's personality."[10] The problem isn't the medical procedure: The problem lies in the patient's perceptions, and while these are not always readily identifiable, they lie at the heart of somatization.

Perception is why the treatment of somatization is typically so frustratingly difficult. The physician argues the symptoms have no clear etiology while the patient argues they are in pain. We are unintentionally at cross-purposes with one another. Of course the symptoms have no clear etiology: They derive from the patient. We have to learn how to approach symptoms as integral, rather than foreign, to the patient as a person. It is for this reason that we regard existential psychotherapy as the most viable treatment approach for working with situational somatization. Existential psychotherapy focuses on the patient's experience and perceptions rather than on the illness per se. In the case of the pre-somatizing patient, it prepares him or her to cope with an existential threat by directly addressing the patient's fears and shoring up other defenses to prevent the regression into somatization. For the patient who has already undergone medical treatment, existential psychotherapy walks the patient through the process of resolving the existential crisis and normalizing his/her experience. In both cases, the therapist is neither a teacher nor coach but an actual participant in the patient's existential struggle.

SOMATIZATION AND EXISTENTIAL PSYCHOTHERAPY

In our current economically driven health care system, psychotherapy has been obliged to become streamlined, and the emphasis is now upon treatments that are brief, symptom-oriented, and inexpensive. For the situational somatizer, this works to our advantage. Very few of the personality types that are somatization-prone have the ego strength to tolerate a great deal of therapeutic probing and most are disinclined to enter therapy in the first place. Consequently, we believe a short-term approach can actually be more effective with this population. At the same time, patients are more likely to complete time-limited therapy because the end is in sight from the beginning. Short-term therapy also allows the practitioner to focus on the issues that are most important to restore patient functioning and avoid becoming sidetracked by extraneous patient concerns.

At this point, the astute reader might argue that CBT or DBT might be better choices for the situational somatizer. After all, there is a great deal of data supporting the use of cognitive-based therapies with medical and psychiatric patients as noted in chapters 7 and 8. First of all, we suggested CBT, CBMT, and DBT for the chronic somatizer because these treatments are designed to assist patients with poorly developed ego structures to learn how to manage their symptoms and become less reliant upon the perception of bodily illness to support daily functioning. The situational somatizer, however, is able to function in ways not generally attainable by the chronic sub-type and, thus, somatization thus serves a defensive, rather than ego-integrative function.

For CBT to be effective, the clinician must deal with the patient's beliefs about illness, pain, dependency, or loss, identify errors in thinking, and help the patient counter these with alternative cognitions. In so doing, the CBT therapist either bypasses the existential concerns that prompt situational somatization or mistakenly communicate that they are unimportant. S/he may also send a clear signal to the patient that their symptoms are based on faulty ways of thinking and, thus, create the conditions for a potential adversarial relationship with the patient. What we want to do is generate trust which will facilitate a therapeutic relationship in which we can work with the patient. In order to accomplish this, we must leave the patient's symptoms alone—at least initially—and instead, treat the existential crisis which underlies symptom production in the first place.

By focusing on the underlying causes of the patient's distress we communicate our acceptance of the patient's description of their condition. Acceptance creates the perception of a safe environment in which the patient can begin to be honest and genuine—with the clinician and, eventually, with themselves. We're not saying the clinician can't use CBT or any other treatment modality, for that matter, with the situational somatizer. From our perspective however, a roundabout approach to the patient's pathology is preferable and particularly, one that is specifically tailored to handling existential issues. Mindful of our earlier comments about the usefulness of a brief therapy model, we believe we act wisely when we employ short-term existential therapy in the treatment of the situational somatizer.

Before we present the details of short-term existential therapy, we would like to add a word of explanation especially for the primarily medical reader. At first glance, it might seem unnecessary to set forth the details of a therapeutic model for the clinician who is not also a psychotherapist. All of our patients, though, confront important existential issues at various stages in the life cycle. Whether we are pediatricians or internists, surgeons or psychiatrists, we are always thrust into the position of dealing with persons in need. When we must explain to a patient that they have cancer or comfort a family which has lost a loved one, it is tremendously advantageous to have the tools of existential therapy at hand. In whatever way we find the words to speak the unspeakable, it is invaluable to have some idea about how we are going to be perceived by the patient. Whether we are just beginning the journey of a physician or anticipate retirement, we too are subject to the same existential concerns and limitations. The hope we seek to offer, we claim for ourselves; the pain we seek to assuage, we must also be willing to embrace.

THE PRACTICE OF EXISTENTIAL PSYCHOTHERAPY

With that said, what do we mean by "existential psychotherapy"? Clearly, it is a psychotherapy model that focuses on issues and concerns that are part and parcel of our existence as human beings. With existential psychotherapy, "each person is viewed as a unique individual human being facing the responsibility for, and finiteness of, his own life in the concrete historical situation of this world. This is different from the usual approach of psychology as an empirical science concerning itself with data and theories that can be generalised."[11] Irvin Yalom defines existential psychotherapy as "a dynamic approach which focuses on concerns that are rooted in an individual's existence."[12] The term "dynamic" is important because existential psychotherapy pays close attention to the interplay of conscious and unconscious perceptions, motivations, and fears that are at work within an individual.

Like other dynamic psychotherapies (Freudian, Jungian, etc.), existential psychotherapy deals with anxiety and psychological defenses. Rather uniquely, however, the existential therapist views anxiety as the result of an individual's encounter with issues of ultimate concern, that is, death, freedom, isolation, and meaninglessness.[13] In fact, these four ultimate concerns are encountered in various ways throughout existential psychotherapy. Psychological defenses are ways of avoiding contact with these ultimate concerns. Besides enabling us to cope with anxiety, defenses allow us to maintain certain beliefs about ourselves which may or may not be exactly true. For example, one of the primary ways we defend ourselves against the awareness of our own mortality is the belief that we are somehow special and "are exempt from biological necessity and that life will not deal with us in the same harsh way it deals with everyone else."[14] In existential therapy, the patient is exposed to the ultimate concerns which are perceived as a threat to existence.

Although the content of each session is determined by the patient, there should be an overall framework which guides the process. A framework differs from a treatment protocol that suggests a formal treatment strategy which designates a series of topics to be covered over a given period of time, perhaps in chronological order. A protocol works fine with behavioral methods where the therapist is as much a teacher as anything else. By "framework" we mean the existential conditions that characterize human experience. These can't be determined in advance like a lesson plan because existential therapy (as does all therapy, when it comes down to it) depends on an organic relationship between therapist and patient. In a very real sense, it is the relationship that heals. In this short-term model, we are talking about ten to twelve weekly sessions with no more than two follow-up sessions at four- to six-week intervals.

In the course of exploring the patient's history, feelings about being in therapy, whatever thoughts or anxieties they may communicate about their condition, the existential issues will surface—this much is predictable. The task of the therapist is to point them out and help the patient work through them, within the limitations of time. Once again, we don't have unlimited resources with which to work and we are typically dealing with patients who would rather be someplace else. This means we may not see the kind of transformation that is possible with long-term therapy, but that's not our goal. Our goal is more specific and near-term, but there can be great worth in that as well.

The content of the sessions, that is, the therapeutic framework, is established by the issues themselves: the existential "facts of life." Briefly, these are uncertainty, interpersonal relationships, time and temporality, the four dimensions of existence, and existential anxiety.[15] Uncertainty refers simply to the unpredictability of life to which the inflexible ego structure of somatizing patients renders them very sensitive. Indeed, as we have frequently noted, the entire lifestyle of the situational somatizer can be viewed as a defense against inconsistency and unpredictability. The formation of interpersonal relationships is, in part, a response to the insecurity that is inherent in existence. From the moment we enter the world, we do so in community. We find solace, strength, and dependability in our interactions with others. For many somatizers, interpersonal relationships may have been a source of insecurity due to poor parenting, divorce, and death. It is almost axiomatic that the therapeutic relationship offers patients a corrective experience which has healing effects.

Time and temporality remind us that no one is exempt from aging. We all pass through fairly predictable stages of development, each marked by the accomplishment of particular tasks. For the situational somatizer, the possibility of illness and disability is heightened by the, at least unconscious, awareness that time is not always a friend and we have promises to keep and miles to go.

The four dimensions of existence relate to our physical, public, private, and spiritual worlds.[16] None of us can escape the limitations of the physical world and the knowledge that death is inevitable. We are social creatures and, barring pathology, we strive to reduce isolation by relating to others. By the exercise of freedom, we establish a self-concept and a sense of self-worth which connects us with our private world. The term "spiritual" represents the search for meaning and the mighty struggle against the fear that who we are and what we do is, ultimately, purposeless.

Existential anxiety is "the emotion that is in the background and rooted in all human existence."[17] The fact of being alive in a world where the unpredictable can occur, results in anxiety that is the common human experience. Existential anxiety is more generalized in the sense that it is not about a particular thing or event. We aren't anxious because its tax time or we have to go to the doctor. We are anxious at a deep, intrapersonal level because we are subject to forces beyond our control and living means being vulnerable.

Humans tend to respond to the conditions of existence in predictable ways. These include the creation of values and systems of behavior, the establishment of polarities, the creation of self-concept and self-esteem, and finally, the freedom to choose. In the face of the inescapable existential limitations of life, we create values and patterns of behavior that make life livable. For example, we value heroism and personal sacrifice which fly in the face of hopelessness. We establish socially acceptable patterns of behavior that maintain order and preserve life. Furthermore, we adopt those values and patterns of behavior for which we are temperamentally suited and these become the basis for much of our social functioning. For example, an individual who believes that one can only live meaningfully by nurturing spirituality, might feel compelled to associate with a religious tradition. Persons who do not conform to this individual's understanding of existence may be considered abnormal, immoral, or heathen.

Polarities are built into all value systems. Good is opposed by evil, beauty by ugliness, normality by abnormality. Persons whose values are dominated by extremes tend to exhibit rigid ego structures as well. Accordingly, exploring the poles of a patient's value system is an extremely important therapeutic technique. The creation of a self-concept and nurturance of self-esteem reflect a patient's overall attitude toward existence. For example, does a person possess a self-concept that is adaptive and shows a positive attitude toward existence or do they imagine themselves as helpless victims and refuse nurturance altogether? Freedom of choice is a sticky subject because we generally admit there are circumstances which limit our choices. The accidents of birth, economics, racial prejudice, and the like, exert controlling influences upon the degree to which freedom of choice can be exercised. Nevertheless, existential therapy affirms that individuals have some ability of self-determination, even if it is only to determine one's attitude toward one's limitations.

The elements of short-term existential therapy are major tools in the therapeutic process. That this is a time-limited therapy stands as a constant reminder to both therapist and patient of the temporary character of the relationship. The "knowledge of ending and separation frequently has the effect of evoking strong emotions, such as the fear of rejection. This can take many forms, including anger, sadness, and relief, all of which can be worked through as (patients) learn to identify their value and coping mechanisms."[18] The expectations of therapist and patient about the outcome of therapy are also important factors to consider. One of the aims of time-limited therapy is for patients to alter their expectations from those that are unrealistic to those that are attainable.[19] This is particularly important for hypernormal and managerial types which are so intent upon controlling their environments. Altering expectations creates flexibility which can help a patient accept the limitations placed upon them by surgical recovery, for example, without having to resort to somatization to "excuse" their perceived weakness. Furthermore, we work toward helping the patient associate dependency with the capacity to trust, where trust creates an environment in which the patient feels comfortable with intimacy without the fear of judgment or condemnation.[20]

One of the remarkable things about therapy is the way it allows a patient's painful relationships, past history, and existential conflicts to be re-created. In short-term existential therapy, patient and therapist re-enact many of the existential conditions of life—time and its ending, the potential for intimacy and trust, the quest for meaning, and the limits of choice. Through this relationship we work to detoxify the fear that drives the patient toward somatization. By addressing the issues that prompt somatization, we generate an environment in which the need to somatize can either be eliminated or at least reduced in intensity.

The following vignette can help illustrate the process of existential psychotherapy. The patient is a 49-year-old Caucasian male who has been employed for a number of years as a computer analyst. By his own admission, he prefers a highly structured and predictable environment and has a proclivity for "obeying the rules." He states these preferences extend to his personal life as well, and he and his wife follow a fairly strict schedule of weekly activities. His checkbook is always balanced and he has low tolerance for persons who do not conform to societal norms. His medical complaint concerns chronic lower back pain secondary to a series of surgeries to correct an injury he sustained in an auto accident. His pain is sufficiently severe as to necessitate his taking an extended leave of absence from work. Post-surgical workups, including an MRI, have revealed no identifiable etiology for the patient's ongoing discomfort and he has only been partially responsive to analgesic medications. Although he is receiving short-term disability income, he and his wife are beginning to feel some financial strain. He claims he is eager to return to work and is frustrated because his pain prevents him from doing so. He reports decreased appetite and libido, disrupted sleep due to physical discomfort, and states he is more irritable lately. His primary care physician has placed him on an antidepressant and he has been referred for psychotherapy.

Therapist (T): So, how can I be of help?

Patient (P): I'm here because my primary care physician thought it might be helpful. I don't know.

T: You aren't sure if coming here will be helpful?

P: I'm not sure if she really understands what I need. She's giving me an antidepressant.

T: Have you been taking it?

P: For a few weeks. It seems to help, I suppose, though I don't know how it's going to make a difference. I need to get back to work. My wife and I are doing ok, but disability isn't going to last forever and I hate sitting around the house.

T: You're concerned about the future?

P: Of course, I'm concerned. I need to work, I hurt all the time, and I can't really sleep. You want to know the last time I slept through the night? It was months ago, before all this started.

T: All this?

P: The surgeries, the medications—pain relief, they call it. May as well be candy. I've been on Darvacet, Percocet, Vicodan—you name it. Works for a while and then, nothing. Now my doctor says it's all in my head. Great.

T: Do you think it's all in your head?

P: Hell, no. I don't know why I see *that* bastard, anyway, for all the good it does. If it was all in my head, would I spend all this money trying to get well? He's just frustrated because he doesn't know what's wrong, so he blames me instead. Now, that's what being a "doctor" gets you.

T: I'm not sure I follow you. You said your PCP prescribed an antidepressant and now you're referring to someone who seems to suggest your pain is imaginary.

P: I see a pain specialist. Really, he's the reason I'm here. My PCP thought it was a good idea, but the pain guy said he'd refer me to another doctor if I didn't get some therapy. I guess he's getting tired of me? (patient smiles nervously)

T: It sounds like coming here isn't entirely your idea and you're doubtful whether or not therapy can make a difference to you.

P: That's exactly what I think. Listen: I was a successful computer analyst for a major corporation. I was head of a department with fifteen other analysts working under me. I was making a very good income. One day I'm broadsided by a guy running a red light. Life is good and I get hit by a minivan. What are the odds? I got out of the car and thought I must be ok—no broken bones, I didn't hit my head. The next day I could hardly get out of bed. I'm not someone who gets sick, so I managed to drag myself to the shower, got dressed, and went to work. I was in pain, sure, but I thought a few Ibuprofens and it would pass. Well, it didn't. The next day was worse, and the day after that, and finally, my wife has to drive me to the doctor. She ordered some tests and sent me to see an orthopedist. He diagnosed me with a spinal injury and said I needed surgery. Two more surgeries after that, and they're telling me I should be doing somersaults, but here I am, instead. I can't work, I can't sleep, and the doctor says I'm imagining it all.

T: Sounds like you've had some losses.

P: Yeah, I've lost some things, including my stupidity. I won't ever trust a doctor again who tells me I'll be up and around in no time, you can count on that.

T: So, you've lost your faith in doctors.

P: I've lost my faith in them and frankly, I don't know who to trust. I mean, can you ever trust anybody completely?

T: Is there anyone you feel you can trust?

P: I told you, I'm not sure anymore. I suppose I trust my wife—I guess. Sometimes I'm not even certain about her.

T: Losing faith is hard; it leaves you feeling somewhat adrift.

P: I hadn't thought of it that way, but that's true: I do feel uncertain. Uncertain and in pain. What a hell of a situation. But what can I do?

T: Lack of certainty; that sounds scary.

P: Not so much scary as it is irritating. I don't like uncertainty, you know. I like things planned and organized. This business of depending on a doctor to tell you something you already know is for the birds.

T: You sound angry. I'm wondering if that's related to your feeling as though things are out of control.

P: Hell, yes, I'm angry! I don't know if control's the problem or not, but like I say, I do like things predictable and all that's predictable for me right now is misery. That's not what I had in mind for my life. I watched my father become an old man right before my eyes. He had arthritis and by the time he was fifty, he could hardly move. When he could walk, it was with a cane. I still have it, by the way. The cane, I mean.

T: Aren't you fifty?

P: (Silence) Forty-nine. What are you saying? That I'm afraid of turning into my father? Is that it? You think this is "Field of Dreams"? (laughs sardonically)

T: It's just curious that you mentioned your father and his disability.

P: Yeah and he got along just fine.

T: I'm not so sure about that. You said that your father could scarcely walk and, even then, only with assistance. He must have been in considerable pain. You have nearly constant pain, you can't sleep, you aren't working, you're irritable, and you're forty-nine. I'm wondering if you aren't concerned that you're going to suffer the same fate as your father.

P: Jesus. You shrinks are all alike. You think that because somebody's having a problem it must because they "hate their father." Listen, for the record, I'm here because my pain doctor said he'd refer me to someone else if I didn't get some therapy. I wasn't sexually abused, my dad didn't beat me, my mother wasn't a prostitute. I had a normal family life and I was doing ok until the damned accident. Now what can you do for me besides sit there and make accusations?

T: I appreciate your honesty. I take it you'd like me to be just as straight with you.

P: Well, that would be a switch. So, you're saying I'm hopeless? I just have to learn to live with "this"?

T: I think we all have to learn to live with things we'd rather live without. Is that what's so painful for you? Thinking you're situation is hopeless?

P: Is it hopeless?

T: I'm not sure, but I don't think "you" are hopeless.

P: What's the difference?

T: The difference is, you're having a difficult time seeing an end to your suffering, but you are much more than your suffering. You're a human being with dreams, ambitions, and the desire to live life fully once again.

P: Right, I'd agree with that, but I still have my pain, and it doesn't go away. If it wasn't for that, I'd be the man you describe.

T: Does your pain make you any less a man?

P: I wonder . . . sometimes I think so. When my son wants me to play soccer with him and then says, "I'm sorry, Dad, I forgot, it's ok. We'll do it when you get better." Do you know what that's like? I know he's disappointed and I can't do anything about it. What kind of father am I? Do you have kids?

T: Yes, I do, and I can only imagine how it must feel when that happens to you.

P: It's awful; I wouldn't wish it on anyone.

T: I have an idea that your experience with the accident, the surgeries, and so forth, have struck at the heart of who you are as a person.

P: Maybe. I don't know. What do you mean?

T: When a person has an experience like yours, they start asking themselves questions they've never asked before. What does it mean for me to be a man? What makes my life worthwhile? What's truly important to me? How can I have hope when all seems lost? Make sense?

P: Yeah, it does, and I've been asking myself those questions. Sometimes it just feels like I'm dead inside. Like I can't feel anything. I must be losing my grip. Am I going crazy?

T: It is like a death. The little deaths we encounter in life remind us, unconsciously, that we are eventually going to have to face death itself. That's what makes loss so powerful and so difficult to bear.

P: I feel dead inside because I'm afraid of dying?

T: Maybe. Maybe you feel dead inside because all the things you've counted on to give you a sense of purpose are "on hold." Your pain is costing you a great deal more than simply lost income. It's costing you the things you hold dear.

P: What do I do? I mean, I just don't know what to do. (sighs, wipes away a tear)

T: The most important thing for you right now is to continue talking about these very things: What matters most to you, what makes life meaningful for you.

P: Yeah, but isn't that going to make me more miserable? Talking about those things just reminds me how much it hurts to be where I am. I don't want to get more depressed.

T: It's been my experience that people become depressed when they ignore the things that matter most to them. Most people are like that, you know. They go through life assuming that everything is pretty much ok. Sure, they have problems like everyone. They have some disappointments and, perhaps, even some losses. But then something happens that strikes at the heart of their sense of personal identity, something that makes them aware that life is unpredictable and bad things happen, sometimes even death. Those experiences can either debilitate or invigorate them. Up until now, you've been feeling pretty debilitated, I would guess. Does that sound right?

P: Yeah, go on.

T: Our task is to help you come to grips with what your experience means. The success of our work depends a great deal on you and how willing you are to be honest with yourself and with me. I promise I will work as diligently as you, I won't pull my punches, and I won't lose hope.

Obviously, this vignette does not represent an entire session with the patient; it has been edited for the sake of brevity and is designed to highlight the value of an indirect approach with a situational patient who is actually a composite figure drawn from the authors' experiences. Notice the therapist validates the patient's perceived pain and debilitation while interpreting his experience in existential terms. No attempt has been made to reframe the patient's comments in terms reflective of psychopathology or the outcome of mistaken beliefs. Instead, the therapist assumes the patient's description genuinely represents the kind of distress one might expect of someone whose life has been abruptly interrupted. By drawing attention to the core issues the patient is facing, the therapist lays the foundation for a therapeutic relationship based on trust and the patient's belief that he is being heard and understood. The element of trust is critical, particularly in view of the fact that the patient claims his faith in healing practitioners has been damaged as a result of unsatisfactory treatment outcomes. Furthermore, he is quite angry because he thinks his medical providers question the veracity of his reports about his pain. His fear that he is "losing his mind" is reality based; he has depended upon the trappings of functionality—work, family, social acceptance—to provide him with both a sense of identity and a sense of normalcy. Presented with real or perceived losses in all of these areas, his coping strategies are severely compromised and he fears he might be "losing his grip." In a real sense, this is true; the terror of madness is hardly imaginary. Under ordinary circumstances, the patient's compulsive personality serves to keep unconscious material from disrupting his daily life. As long as he is in control, as long as life is predictable, he feels "sane." Remove those critical elements and a pre-psychotic character structure begins to emerge and he begins to experience symptoms which we would identify as mildly paranoid. Somatization entered the picture to shore up his personality but its consequences have created a great deal of misery and, despite his contention that he has come to therapy to placate his "pain doctor," he is desperately afraid he will never recover. For him, this is tantamount to madness. In short, our patient is appropriately fearful of ceasing to exist in any meaningful way.

One of the inherent difficulties we encounter with the existential approach is the heterogeneous nature of its theory and practice. In a sense there isn't a single existential psychotherapy; there are as many as there are practitioners. The absence of procedural guidelines renders empirical validation problematic. The ease with which CBT can be manualized helps explain why it has received so much research attention. Keshen suggests a way in which existential psychotherapy can be formulated in order to facilitate validation of its outcomes. The clinician begins by an evaluation of the patient's symptoms and employment of "purpose substitutes" (substance abuse, workaholism, illness, etc.) to avoid confrontation of questions related to personal meaning and truth. The clinician then develops an existential formulation of the pathology relative to the pursuit of "authentic purpose," which Keshen defines as "anything one has a genuine love or interest in."[21] The next step involves discovery of the patient's authentic purpose. One way this can be pursued is to ask such questions such as, what would you do with your life if you were diagnosed with a terminal illness. The final steps involve facilitating the pursuit of authentic purpose and discontinuation of purpose substitutes.[22]

Applying Keshen's organization to our clinical vignette, the patient's symptoms are represented by physical pain and depression. The existential formulation could draw from themes to which our patient has alluded: Vulnerability and dependency, death anxiety and the loss of functioning, unpredictability and the loss of control, interpersonal relationships and the loss of faith/trust, disability, and the loss of self-esteem. Each one of these could easily provide the material for many hours of therapy, but therapist and patient need to establish guidelines that limit their work and decide where the patient's primary concerns lie. Accordingly, if we formulate our patient's situation in existential terms we might say that he has substituted a compulsive preoccupation with structure and responsibility for a sense of authentic purpose. Instead of confronting his fears of meaninglessness, he has resorted to somatization as a defense against ego disintegration. Although the vignette did not describe the process of discovery of the patient's authentic purpose, its pursuit and discontinuation of purpose substitutes, those could constitute the next steps.

The resolution of somatization depends largely on the patient. Ego strength is not unilateral in the situational population any more than it is among chronic somatizers. Some patients may experience something approaching complete symptom relief while others may require more time. Clinical judgment and the patient's commitment to therapy are the critical factors in this determination. Evaluation of the residual presence of somatization might be achieved by using screening tools such as PRIME-MD or the Paindex® test.[23] Ideally, one of these instruments would be employed at the beginning of therapy and again at termination to help measure progress.

There are some important considerations when contemplating existential psychotherapy with the situational patient. We have to evaluate ego strength and one of the ways that's accomplished is by observing the patient's response to the existential formulation of their primary concerns. Can they accept these comments as accurate reflections of their experience or do they seem confused and deny their validity? Is there any indication of openness to the therapist? Does the patient voice willingness and motivation to try a new approach to their situation? We also have to look at their premorbid functioning, the quality of social supports, and the presence of psychiatric comorbidity.

From our perspective, the situational patient most suited to existential psychotherapy is one who voices concerns about guilt, failure, and loss and its associated feelings. The autocratic-managerial type, for example, who complains that she has always valued her independence and strength of character and now feels as though her body has failed her, is already expressing an existential theme. Or the patient in our clinical vignette who laments feeling guilty over his inability to play ball with his son. When patients can communicate this kind of emotional awareness they indicate they have the insight to see how their illness impacts them at multiple levels. The presence of situational somatization alone is insufficient to indicate the appropriateness of existential psychotherapy. The patient has to demonstrate some capacity for relating and if this is absent, for whatever reason, one should consider a behavioral or pharmacological option.

Therapy is less about where the therapist wants to take the patient as it is about how far the patient is willing to go and this is determined by ego strength. There is always the danger of Level III contents interfering with therapy. If the patient has a great deal of paranoid masochism, for example, the greatest concern is the absence of trust, and this reflects fear of an unpredictable universe. The clinician must be realistic about the patient's capability; it might be better to do too little than attempt too much. It's entirely possible to probe beyond the limits of ego strength and trigger decompensation. It is for this reason that existential psychotherapy should be undertaken by the psychiatrist or psychologist who has developed considerable clinical judgment resulting from considerable clinical experience. The reader should not assume that simply because they've read and digested this chapter they are completely qualified to lead any situational patient through a course of therapy. Practicing existential therapy with a vulnerable population like the one we describe is very different from attending a conference on a behavioral modality and then using the manual as a stepwise guide. There is a great deal more uncertainty, ambiguity, and risk involved. Working with these patients is demanding and requires emotional engagement on the part of the therapist. We would strongly suggest the clinician become completely familiar with the practice of existential psychotherapy as well as the process of somatization before proceeding to see patients. Furthermore, as in any therapy, supervision is a valuable tool to have available and particularly so with somatization.

It is not easy to direct therapy toward an existential focus. In actuality, it is much easier to become embroiled in the patient's physical complaints because that's the direction the patient's defenses want to take. Resistant individuals would like nothing more than for the therapist to collude with them and avoid the issues that prompt somatization. Avoidance drives the patient to try to derail the conversation and redirect its focus onto bodily discomfort. It also allows the therapist to sidestep the possibility of incurring the patient's wrath with accusations of empathic failure. More important, addressing existential concerns forces the therapist to become aware of his/her own mortality, vulnerability, and the like. If s/he has managed to sidestep these concerns in their own life, it is going to be very difficult to communicate effectively with the patient. This is not to say we must have experienced similar stressors as the patient, but it does mean that we must endeavor to become conscious of our own responses to the conditions of existence. The truth be told, we are going to re-experience many of these same conditions in the course of therapy with a situational patient.

If we are active at all in therapy, we may find our own experiences surface in the guise of the patient's. The reader will identify this process as countertransference. Unlike Freud, however, we do not regard countertransference as an element which intrinsically interferes with therapy.[24] Instead, we believe our emotional responses to the patient provide critical information about the depth of the patient's struggle and its resolution.[25] For example, Margaret Little observes:

> Consciously, and surely to a great extent unconsciously too, we all want our patients to get well, and we can identify readily with them in their desire to get well, that is with their ego. But unconsciously, we tend to identify also with the patient's super-ego and id, and thereby with him, in any prohibition on getting well, and in his wish to stay ill and dependent, and by so doing we may slow down his recovery. Unconsciously we may exploit a patient's illness for our own purposes, both libidinal and aggressive, and he will quickly respond to this.[26]

If we read between the lines of Little's Freudian terminology, we realize that patients are split between a conscious desire to get well and an unconscious inclination to remain ill. We see this in situational patients regularly. When we permit ourselves to avoid existential pain, we communicate a powerful message to our patients; that is, existential issues really are too dangerous and threatening to be examined. If we aren't willing to confront the heart of the matter, can we expect anything else from our patients?

Ultimately, this is why we are so disinclined to use cognitive or behavioral therapies with situational patients. By focusing on the patient's thinking processes or dysfunctional beliefs about illness, both therapist and patient enable one another to avoid the hard facts of life. Situational somatizers rightly perceive themselves as locked in a struggle which seems overwhelming. Issues of existence can be truly overwhelming, which is why we all go to such lengths to ignore them whenever possible. In order to achieve the kind of engagement that is absolutely necessary to resolve or at least relieve the drive toward somatization, the therapist must become a partner in the patient's existential struggle. While the patient's illness experience may represent a perceptual error, the underlying fears of isolation, death, and extinction are real.

Treatment options for chronic and situational somatizers aren't as complicated as we have generally thought. The problem is more a matter of our own misconceptions regarding the nature of somatization and the attendant frustration which results from expecting our patients to fit inside a box that is simply the wrong shape to begin with. Our situational patients can provide us with an opportunity to explore the critical issues of life that possess the power to debilitate and enliven. Working with both chronic and situational patients demands creativity, compassion, and self-awareness. By tapping into these resources, we experience our potential to grow, not only as professionals, but also as human beings.

Chapter Ten

Psychopharmacology and Somatization

One factor that we must examine is the use of psychoactive medications in the treatment of somatization. Certainly one should be aware that patients who are inclined to resist the suggestion that their symptoms are psychosomatic can also be expected to resist taking psychoactive medications for the same reason. Nevertheless, providing what we believe to be viable and effective (where possible, evidence-based) treatment options for symptom relief, if not cure, is our duty as physicians. The earlier chapters in this work attend to rational and non-pharmacological approaches to patients with somatoform-related problems. In large measure, we presume that these patients have either decided or been persuaded to place themselves in the qualified hands of a therapist skilled in one or more of the modalities we have described. The question remains, however, is there a role for psychopharmacology in the treatment of somatization and if so, which medications may be regarded as effective and are there any guidelines for the would-be prescriber? The answer to the first question is frequently as elusive as the one to the second. Furthermore, clinical wisdom on the subject tends to be anecdotal. Pardon us for beating a dead horse, but the truth of the matter is, somatization and somatoform disorders simply have not received the kind or degree of attention devoted to their cohorts in physical medicine or the major classifications of the DSM series. Hopefully, this will change over time as consultation-liaison psychiatry continues to come into its own as a field of critical inquiry. It should be noted that this presentation is not intended as an exhaustive exploration of the pharmaceutical options available to the practitioner. There are a number of excellent resources to which one can turn for this kind of thing. We feel we can make our best contribution by discussing some of the problems we face in prescribing medications for this population and pointing the clinician in the direction of effective options.

One of the most pressing issues facing the prescriber with the somatizing patient is polypharmacy. Many of those with somatoform complaints who rely on family physicians, consultation-liaison psychiatrists, neurologists, and the like for medical care have been exposed to an increasing variety of drugs—in some cases, for years. Similarly, in the relevant physician's hands are a variety of choices. In consultation with the patient, test results may show minor abnormalities or some unusual symptoms suggesting further medical approaches, and both patient and physician are of the belief that there is "something out there" that should help. Sometimes there is, but not often. The pursuit of the ever-elusive treatment is the source of much frustration as we've noted repeatedly. Added to this, we have patients with long histories of somatic problems with or without vestigial justifications, who end up on polypharmacy; so do patients with schizophrenia or major depression, but in these cases, some legitimate improvement is likely. In somatization, we essentially have a population prone to modularizing their symptoms, taking multiple drugs, still hoping for a new and better potion or diagnosis and having acquired some new symptoms from the drugs they are taking.

A somatizing patient may be maintained, for example, on a benzodiazepine for anxiety, an SSRI for depression, a sedative atypical antipsychotic (e.g., quetiapine), an anticonvulsant (e.g., valproic acid), plus an anti-Parkinson's drug for locomotor side effects, urecholine for dry mouth, and a beta blocker for cardiac irregularities, plus whatever else has been prescribed for cardiac or endocrine-related conditions. The senior medical author relates how he has been brought in as a consultant in such cases and been forced to make quick decisions based on the patient's memory of which pills did what, coupled with voluminous medical records, most of which record changes in medication but rarely mention whey they were begun in the first place. Tracking down a patient's list of medications, as well as their understanding of them, can be a knotty problem. And because patients are inclined to continue medications "because the doctor told me to," in some cases it is difficult to determine whether their condition has been improved or exacerbated by polypharmacy. The senior medical author notes that, in his more than fifty years in the field of psychiatry, he can recall occasional small studies where a drug (e.g., propranolol) masked phobic symptoms so well, for example, that when the drugs were removed, the patient retained the full, original phobia.

The idea of a drug holiday has certain appeal because it's often unclear to what extent the patient's complaints represent physical distress, personality structure, or the miracles of modern chemistry. But patient preference figures into the equation and drugs such as benzodiazepines, opiates, and some atypical antipsychotics that make one feel better rapidly (minutes to hours as opposed to weeks) are often held onto tenaciously. One rarely sees a somatizing patient who insists on keeping their sertraline active when its effects may be less dramatic, albeit more helpful long-term, than hydrocodone. So, do we suggest behavioral therapies to help ease patients off medications in order to get an idea of what we're dealing with? At least one Boston hospital has used such therapies to good effect. In most cases, however, it seems that psychological therapies coupled with medications produce rather different, but complimentary, effects. Given the relative expense, rebuilding difficulties, and scarcity of good therapists, one wonders if Paul Meehl's cynical view doesn't hold: only 10 percent of therapists are good at managing medical patients and only 20 percent of patients are likely to respond. The chance of a "good" patient and a "good" therapist coming together yields an odd guess of about 5 percent of all patients doing well. Still, unless medically necessary, polypharmacy can complicate a clinical picture to the point where one begins to wonder if it hurts as much as it helps.

Ultimately, the real problem in drug treatment, at least so far as it appears to us, is the fact that we really don't know how to treat somatization as a process. We're comfortable talking about it as a correlative phenomenon in major psychiatric disorders, but not so much as the underlying culprit that presents in somatoform disorders. It has been the authors' collective contention from the first chapter that somatization is an interior process of disturbed ego functioning that manifests itself in a chronic or situational manner. Pretty much the closest the literature gets to this is in the case of drug trials that identify patients with Undifferentiated-type Somatoform Disorder, and these aren't generally the primary focus of the study—there are exceptions, of course.[1]

Very possibly the difficulty lies in classification. We seem to be uncertain about identifying what constitutes diagnosable somatization and tend to fall back onto somatic complaints associated with other psychiatric disorders or functional somatic syndromes. Whether for the convenience of billing or out of the need for operable and definable syndromes for the sake of research, it's safe to say we tend to err on the side of what we already know. If we take a cohort of depressed patients with physical pain complaints and run them through an antidepressant trial, we're really working from the premise that physical pain can be secondary to depression. Patients who respond positively with relief of depression and fewer physical symptom complaints are telling us, in effect, what we believe we already know. Because we aren't certain how to identify and/or classify the "pure" somatizer, s/he gets relegated to the periphery. Yet, ironically, this is generally the type of patient commonly seen in the primary care setting.

We've stated previously how we tend to diagnose conditions for which we have established treatments. In essence, it is sometimes simpler for the practitioner to look for and diagnose somatic complaints in the presence of depression or anxiety. The patient seems depressed and anxious, meets most of the criteria for a diagnosis, wants treatment, and it makes sense to go after horses rather than zebras, despite the fact that it might be the zebras causing the problem. In short, we've either approached the subject from the standpoint of the biochemical dysfunction, that is, is it related to a dysfunction in serotonergic, dopaminergic, or GABA-related neurotransmission, or from the perspective of what's taking place in the patient; that is, if there is depression or anxiety, we treat *that* as the primary condition. When we talk about types of drugs, therefore, we have to admit that, to a certain extent, our choices are dictated by our theoretical orientation. Is somatization adjunctive to a mood disturbance, body delusion, or an anxiety process, and if so, that decision dictates our inclination to make certain choices, to reach for one drug and not another on our mental drug cabinet. Bearing in mind, however, that we're addressing ego deficits, in which case we're saying medication makes therapy possible. How can our prescribing practices support psychological therapies designed to improve coping skills, reduce patient suffering, and reduce doctor visits and utilization costs? In essence, the question becomes how can the clinician help alleviate frontal lobe dysfunction?

The evidence helps us a little, at least insofar as it points to agents that have shown some efficacy in clinical trials. Unfortunately, it doesn't provide us with guidelines or an algorithm. But among clinicians familiar with somatizing patients, we suspect to hear a huge collective sigh of relief that there are some agents that are promising. Selecting among them is another thing, which we will get to shortly.

Generally, antidepressant treatment of somatoform complaints shows a moderate to fairly good treatment response. In a rather large meta-analysis, O'Malley et al. found that patients with functional somatic syndromes who received selective serotonin reuptake inhibitors and, particularly, tricyclic antidepressants, were three times more likely to improve than with a placebo.[2] A study of prescribing habits of consultation-liaison psychiatrists by Smith et al. shows a preference for using antidepressants with psychosomatic illness.[3] Among the SSRIs with somatization/somatoform disorders, there is data available on trials of fluoxetine with hypochondriasis,[4] Body Dysmorphic Disorder,[5] dermatologic conditions,[6] major depression with somatic complaints,[7] and chronic tension headache.[8] Of particular interest is a study of fluoxetine in the treatment of Undifferentiated Somatoform Disorder.[9] In this open label study of forty-five patients, fluoxetine was compared to sertraline, with each drug showing a significant decline in somatic symptoms.[10] However, one study indicates the severity of physical symptoms tends to be a limiting factor in fluoxetine response for Major Depressive Disorder; that is, the presence and severity of psychic and somatic anxiety predicted an increased likelihood of non-response to fluoxetine.[11]

Sertraline has been tried in patients with chronic subjective dizziness with good outcomes related to symptom relief.[12] In a study of 267 patients with Premenstrual Dysphoric Disorder, 31 of which were diagnosed with comorbid OCD, anxiety, and somatoform disorders, Alpay and Turhan found that sertraline administered continuously, rather than intermittently, tended to produce positive outcomes as well as increased patient compliance.[13] As have other SSRIs, sertraline has been associated with treatment for PTSD with comorbid somatization.

Paroxetine has received some attention in the literature. One case study exists in which a patient diagnosed with Somatization Disorder was started on paroxetine at 10 mg qday, titrated to 40 mg qday, achieved a positive response and was discharged on 30 mg qday for maintenance therapy.[14] In addition, a study of patients with Irritable Bowel Syndrome with somatization tried on paroxetine and psychotherapy showed a response comparable to non-somatizing IBS patients.[15] Paroxetine has been studied in patients with non-cardiac chest pain with positive results.[16] A comparative study of paroxetine with citalopram has been tried in Primary Movement Disorder with conversion symptoms indicating SSRIs may be useful in treating such conditions.[17]

According to Croom et al., mirtazapine shows promise in the treatment of Undifferentiated Somatoform Disorder.[18] A study of pre- and post-menopausal women showed positive results in reduction of somatic symptoms with mirtazapine and a 12-week parallel trial of venlafaxine and mirtazapine in Undifferentiated Somatoform Disorder showed comparable, and positive outcomes.[19] There is some data indicating the serotonin-norepinephrine reuptake inhibitor nefazodone has potential for treating patients with diagnosed Hypochondriasis or Somatization Disorder. [20]

Among newer agents, escitalopram has been studied in Multisomatoform Disorder in a double-blind, placebo controlled trial involving fifty-one patients.[21] The outcome indicated escitalopram was superior to placebo and associated with lower symptom scores, increased response and remission rates, and improved functioning.[22] A randomized double-blind comparison of reboxetine and citalopram has shown comparable results between noradrenergic and serotonergic antidepressants, suggesting citalopram to have a moderate analgesic effect in patients with DSM Pain Disorder.[23]

As far as naturopathic remedies are concerned, in a randomized, multicenter, placebo-controlled trial of 151 patients with Somatization Disorder, Undifferentiated Somatoform Disorder, and somatoform autonomic dysfunction, Volz et al. determined hypericum extract to be superior to placebo in reducing somatic anxiety even after splitting depressed from non-depressed patients.[24] In view of the fact that studies of major depression have not tended to show a statistical difference between St. John's Wart and placebo, Volz et al. suggests a different biological process may be at work in the case of somatoform disorders. While there is evidence that treatment with an SSRI reduces hypothalamus-pituitary-adrenal axis activity in mood-disordered patients, in the Volz et al. study, hypericum extract L1 160 seemed to increase activity along this axis.[25] The authors speculate that HPA axis activity might be inversely regulated in some forms of depression, especially of the melancholic type and somatoform disorders, and St. John's Wart may have a specific biological action to normalize somatoform symptoms.[26]

Overall, clinicians like antidepressants, particularly SSRIs, because they have relatively benign side-effect profiles, especially as compared to the TCAs, and tend to be well-tolerated. For example, Keeley et al. found in a study of 1,000 patients that somatizing patients were more inclined to adhere to antidepressant treatment, particularly when the study controlled for conversion symptoms, suggesting somatization may represent personality states amenable to antidepressant therapy.[27] In a meta-analysis of ninety-four studies, O'Malley et al. determined antidepressant therapy for unexplained symptoms and syndromes to be generally superior to placebo.[28] Hurtz points out that, when somatization co-occurs with PTSD, medications that are considered effective for trauma should coincidentally be effective for somatization.[29] It should be noted, however, that there is some evidence that suggests improvement in somatic symptoms, at least in depressed patients, tends to occur within the first month of treatment, then plateau with minimal resolution in subsequent months.[30] If it is the case that these symptoms are, in fact, representative of somatization as we have discussed throughout this volume, it's not terribly surprising that symptom relief would have a natural ceiling. Patients who rely on somatization for ego support are only going to improve so much before the mind-body connection kicks in and we're back at the starting gate, or at least pretty close.

TCAs have a history of use in the treatment of chronic pain syndromes and we see dual action antidepressants (venlafaxine, duloxetine) frequently prescribed for depressed patients with pain symptoms on the premise that descending serotonergic and noradrenergic pathways are implicated in the generation of painful physical sensations.[31] A recent meta-analysis, however, has thrown some doubt on the analgesic effect of duloxetine.[32] Additional studies are needed to confirm or disconfirm the usefulness of duloxetine for painful symptoms associated with depression.

As noted earlier, some clinicians are inclined to view somatization, depression, and anxiety as more or less coexisting conditions requiring a more unified treatment approach.[33] Henningsen et al. discuss the potential for treating pain, depression, and anxiety as overlapping conditions to aid in etiological and treatment decisions.[34] But in a 2005 study of somatosensory amplification in depressed and fibromyalgia patients, Sayer, Barsky, and Gulec found that while antidepressant therapy certainly improved mood and somatic symptoms among depressed patients, they did not seemed to have similar effect on pain associated with fibromyalgia, despite the fact that these patients, too, experienced alleviation of their depressive symptoms.[35] At the same time, Hand et al., in a relatively small study of diffuse esophageal spasm, eight of nine patients achieved symptom relief on an antidepressant.[36] The point we wish to make is, despite evidence pointing to the utility of antidepressant therapy in the treatment of somatization and somatoform disorders, we're still not in a position to speak in absolutes. We certainly can't say one drug is better than the others nor can we say with any certainty that antidepressants will work consistently outside the rather artificial parameters of a clinical trial.

There seems to be less information, generally speaking, regarding the use of mood stabilizing or anticonvulsants in somatoform disorders. Maurer et al. describe a single case report of a patient with somatoform Pain Disorder comorbid with major depression who, having failed to obtain relief with antidepressants and carbamazepine, achieved symptom relief of both conditions with gabapentin.[37] Garvia-Campayo and Sanz-Carrillo detail an open study of twenty-nine patients with Somatization Disorder and pain as the predominant symptom, treated with gabapentin adjunctive to their normal medication regimen (antidepressants, neuroleptics, benzodiazepines).[38] They report significant improvement with the exception of scales relating to anxiety and depression. Stahl has discussed the use of pregabalin and gabapentin as $\alpha_2\delta$ ligands at voltage-gated sodium channels in the treatment of chronic pain.[39] Pregabalin is an analogue of gabapentin that is under FDA investigation for the treatment of chronic pain as well as epilepsy and anxiety.[40] According to Stahl, these ligands "decrease neurotransmitter release from the presynaptic neuron, which presumably leads not only to anticonvulsant actions but to anxiolytic and antineuralgic (chronic pain reducing) actions."[41] So, it appears gabapentin is showing some promise, at least as far as pain symptoms are concerned, and we await the results (hopefully) of double-blind, placebo-controlled studies to give us additional information to go on.

Benzodiazepines are among the most frequently prescribed medications in Japan for the treatment of psychosomatic illness, but given the high proportion of comorbid Axis-II diagnoses with somatization, the potential for addiction and abuse renders this class of medication less than optimal, at least long-term.

The use of atypical antipsychotic medications, that is, olanzapine, clozapine, risperidone, ziprazidone, aripiprazole, and quetiapine, in the treatment of somatization seems to be relatively new territory. Although studies have been done with olanzapine in hypochondriacal psychosis, for example, a Pubmed search reveals no specific references to the study of atypical antipsychotics with somatization proper.[42] We see them used in Conversion Disorder, as adjunctive treatments in Body Dysmorphic Disorder, and delusional conditions such as Delusional Parisitosis.[43] Off-label usage of atypical antipsychotics by internists in private practice has shown some effectiveness in reducing somatization-related anxiety, but this evidence remains anecdotal.[44] Curiously, depressed patients seem to respond more rapidly to treatment when antidepressant medication is augmented with an atypical antipsychotic.[45] Some have argued that this effect is due to the tendency of patients to under-report psychotic symptoms, but others have suggested this indicates that atypical antipsychotics may act at neural sites which serve as targets of antidepressants, thus improving antidepressant response.[46] This line of thinking implies that atypicals may thus have a broader application than strictly the treatment of psychosis. The practical use of atypical antipsychotics in somatoform disorders obviously awaits further study, but we believe it is strongly warranted. Of course, risk-benefit analysis must be considered. While atypical antipsychotics typically demonstrate a lower incidence of extra-pyramidal symptoms, tardive dyskinesia, and neuroleptic malignant syndrome than is observed with traditional antipsychotics (e.g., haloperidol), this does not completely eliminate the need for careful monitoring. In addition, the problem of weight gain reported with most atypical antipsychotics, raising the concern for diabetes, necessitates educating patients in good nutritional habits. Bearing these issues in mind, the pre-psychotic ego structure of somatizing patients, as well as their tendency to misperceive the nature of somatic symptoms, certainly renders treatment with an atypical antipsychotic coupled with psychotherapy an interesting proposition.

As a side note, one might wonder about the potential for using ECT in refractory patients. There is little in the literature aside from typical references to depression, Bipolar Disorder, psychosis, and the like and what is there doesn't look promising. In a review article concerning ECT for geriatric patients, Zorumski et al. notes ECT seems less effective for depression secondary to somatization.[47] In a study of unipolar depressed patients, Rasmussen et al. found that somatic anxiety and hypochondriasis negatively correlated with positive ECT response among less severely depressed patients and concluded their somatic anxiety was likely a variant of Somatoform Disorder. Among severely depressed patients, however, somatic complaints were unrelated to the outcome of ECT.[48] Beyond these references, a Pubmed search reveals little else besides one each to ECT and conversion disorders and ECT in hypochondriasis.[49] Interestingly, Fink suggests loss of personal memories post-ECT might be best described as a somatoform condition.[50] In any case, it is fairly easy to imagine a population that tends to be as psychologically phobic as most somatizers seem to be, being resistant to the idea of receiving ECT. Still, among patients who are unable to respond to any pharmacotherapy, psychotherapy, or combination thereof, ECT might be an option, depending on comorbidity and the severity of symptoms.

Ultimately, when it comes down to prescribing for somatizing patients, we're not exactly in a comfortable position. The truth is, we really don't have a large body of convincing evidence that gives us a great deal of assurance about the decisions we're making. In more or less specific cases such as hypochondriasis or fibromyalgia, this is less problematic, but for Somatization Disorder, Undifferentiated Somatoform Disorder, Somatoform Disorder NOS, and the underlying process of somatization itself, the ground is less certain. Clinicians who feel compelling treatment decisions should be evidence based may find things even more troublesome. For one thing, the data we have in hand seems to indicate any antidepressant is more or less as good as another. We don't have much to go on with anticonvulsants, and antipsychotics are nearly anyone's guess. In a real sense, we're still in the position of having to rely heavily on experience and clinical judgment. As a consequence, the clinician who is, presumably, most familiar with the individual somatizer in the first place has to evaluate the patient and make an appropriate determination to some degree without the safety net of clearly established, evidence-based guidelines. Some may actually find this state of affairs rather refreshing for the very fact that it requires creative thinking and problem-solving techniques, the very thing that drew many of us to careers in medicine in the first place. Accordingly, the entire present volume is designed to prepare the prescriber to manage the ambiguity of working with an inherently ambiguous and ambivalent population under circumstances that are challenging and in a state of change.

So, what to do? Well, as we've suggested, the "magic bullet" is just as elusive for the prescriber as it is for the patient. The typical course is probably to begin with an SSRI antidepressant, at least as far as compliance, tolerability, and adverse events are concerned. If the patient is nonresponsive at the initial dose and titration doesn't help, we know from experience with other psychiatric syndromes a second drug within the same class has a good likelihood of being effective. If not, then we have to decide whether to switch to a serotonergic-noradrenergic type or augment with an antipsychotic or switch to an anticonvulsant. Mindful of what we've said in previous chapters, the clinician will do well to carefully evaluate the patient for ego deficits and allow their overall level of functioning to be a guiding principle. In some cases, for example, a low dose of atypical antipsychotic may be worth trying instead of an antidepressant simply because it's clear a bit of "ego glue" is more likely to be effective and less anxiety provoking for the patient than waiting for an antidepressant response that may be slow in coming, if it comes at all. Previous poor outcomes with an SSRI as well as comorbidity will naturally influence one's initial choices. It's important to remember, even if the clinician is successful in resolving depression in a known somatizer, the role of somatization in the patient's character structure may result in an incomplete resolution of somatic symptoms. The latter should not be taken as an indicator of treatment failure, but rather as revelatory of the fact that we're dealing with a chronic somatizer and a psychotherapy referral should be considered within the context of our earlier discussions.

Now, assuming the clinician has decided upon psychotropic therapy, the question becomes, how do you get a patient to take psychiatric medications for conditions they believe are entirely somatic? We are convinced the answer lies in the doctor-patient relationship. As with any sort of pharmacotherapy, compliance is dependent on a variety of factors including the patient's expectation of symptom relief, frequency of dosage, the doctor's confidence in the efficacy of the medication and, above all, the patient's belief that the doctor has their best interests at heart. A treatment alliance with somatizing patients is difficult to achieve and even more difficult to maintain. Nevertheless, we would argue that a supportive relationship with the patient has the greatest likelihood of bringing about medication compliance, even with psychotropics, with this patient population. It's a difficult task, making effective treatment decisions for a difficult patient, but that's where the challenge lies and it's worthy of our best efforts.

Chapter Eleven

Death or Transformation

While assembling the chapter sequence of the present volume, it occurred to us that we were actually developing the theme of *an existential perspective on somatization.* Throughout our work, we have focused on a discussion of basic personality factors such as progressive disorganization and multilevel ambivalence. We have also addressed the creative existential aspects of the phenomenon of the bodily transformation of perception, impression, and expression in the patient's experience. These are not only essential for understanding existentialism but also for clarifying the emergence of somatization. To understand the corollary of existential transformation and the development of somatization, it is helpful to compare and contrast these constructs. Existential transformation refers to the conscious and positive resolution of mental conflict in a manner which results in, and reinforces, individual creativity. In somatization, unresolved conflict is displaced in an unconscious, negative regression which results in physical symptom formation. Existential transformation leads to growth and the development of more integrative mental processes, while somatization results in a loss of internal balance and a diminished capacity for adjusting to change. Perceptual distortion reinforces the misperception of interior reality resulting in an exclusively physical expression of selfhood. In the process of existential transformation, psychological experience is contained within one's interior reality. Although psychological experience can be projected outwardly in the expression of love, empathy, and similar emotions, ultimately, it continues to dwell within the self. Likewise, in the case of unconscious regression, mental conflict remains within the self but its source has been altered; it is no longer psychological but physiological. Once again, this process *continues in the self.* The similarity between these two processes can best be described as the dynamics of inner resolution, one positive and the other negative. Creative transformation is the essential attitude of existential resolution while somatization is the defense against ego death resulting from the nightmare of psychosis.

Whether processed consciously or not, existential concerns are the common property of human beings. Although values will differ according to individual perspective, we humans are united by our basic life concerns, such as raising children, confronting mortality, and achieving fulfillment. Furthermore, the potential for the creative transformation of our life experiences forms a basic existential frame of reference. Within this framework, all perceptual attitudes which preserve and stimulate transformation can be considered as positive and life-affirming postulates. Those perceptions that repress or dampen creative transformation can be considered as negative postulates.[1] We understand each human being to possess a teleological focus; that is, the drive and desire to bring about the transformation of experience that ultimately results in growth and wholeness. Out of our own individual history and heritage, we all possess the capacity to create a new pattern of living. Factors that inhibit this potential include fixation and psychosis.[2] We've talked about fixation in the sense of becoming "stuck" in one's experience of ambivalence, and we've described psychosis in terms of the end result of progressive disorganization. Regressive processes such as these inhibit creative development and result in stilted and rigid personality patterns. Ironically, despite the fact that somatization prevents growth in the healthy ego, it also seems to serve a positive function insofar as it arrests the disintegration associated with progressive disorganization.

Wolff points out three additional postulates that we believe specifically relate to somatization. The first of these is the existential postulate of equilibrium. Growth and development proceed in balanced and successive stages; disturbances in one area tend to produce compensatory changes in other areas to preserve homeostasis.[3] The second is the existential postulate of dynamics. The individual is a unity; whatever disturbs a part also disturbs the whole. Rigidity and the tendency to split off and repress parts of one's individuality interfere with the dynamic process of growth.[4] The third postulate is that of transformation. Whenever the process of transformation is arrested, the creative process begins to disintegrate.[5] In somatization, there is a decided absence of balance in ego functioning. We observe this, for example, in situational somatizers who handle the demands of daily life fairly well until presented with a crisis of existential proportions. It's as though nearly all of their ego strength is devoted to managing the mundane side of life and there is simply nothing left for dealing with illness or mortality. In the healthy ego, life stressors produce a shift that allows the individual to flexibly navigate life circumstances, resulting in psychological equilibrium.

Particularly in the existential postulate of dynamics, we find disruption in the relationship between somatizing patients and their psychosomatic relationship. In other words, these individuals seem hardly aware that mind and body constitute a unity. Because of this factor, it is understandable how difficult it must be for them to grasp how psychological disturbance can lead to physiological symptoms. The absence of growth and ego development we typically observe in these patients is the direct consequence of splitting off their ambivalence and concentrating their distress in somatic symptoms. Vaillant describes splitting as a defense against affective ambivalence that assigns all of one's good feelings toward one person, and all the bad ones to a scapegoat.[6] In actuality, most persons restrict splitting to the realm of the imagination. Like Walter Mitty, we read about the lifestyles of the rich and famous and imagine ourselves behaving in ways that are free and adventurous. The reality, however, is we get up every day, go to work, and try to conduct our lives with integrity. Splitting takes a world that is appropriately gray and separates it into "all black and all white, and the individual is left divided against himself or herself."[7]

While we are most familiar with splitting as a defense used by patients with Borderline Personality Disorder, we encounter it with the somatizing patient, especially in the doctor-patient relationship. The clinicians who have failed to provide symptomatic relief are the "bad guys" while the new clinician is the "good guy." This kind of unconscious social contract allows the patient to maintain his or her self-image as the "suffering innocent" and shift responsibility for illness management to the clinician. Whenever the process of creative transformation is blocked by splitting, denial of the mind-body interface, or poor ego development, we find patients "stuck" in the process of somatization and unable to grow. We could use the example of a rabbit attempting to cross the road in front of oncoming traffic. The rabbit's first response is to freeze; then, seeing the approaching tire, he tries to turn back and run for home. Immediately, he spies the other tire and is forced to do the one thing he'd rather *not* do, turn and run at breakneck speed in his original direction.

Somehow we often tend to regress in the face of life's oncoming crises when, in reality, our best hope is to move forward and risk the danger. The healthy ego does not remain in the regressed state, but eventually comes to its senses and faces the task at hand. The somatizer essentially goes to ground; that is, s/he makes the regressive move and argues, often convincingly, that her or his bodily symptoms prevent them from doing otherwise. It isn't that these individuals do not wish to take the risks associated with life, but that they can't. Somatization provides both the means and the justification for truncating the process of creative transformation.

Instead of going through the process of becoming a whole self with a genuine awareness of one's abilities and limitations, somatizers establish a fictional identity based on the avoidance of internal problems which have their origin either in past experience or the present situation. Rather than searching for the solution to existential dilemmas within oneself, the somatizer identifies with fictitious characters and life becomes like a daydream. The analytical task of existential psychotherapy is to unravel and dissolve these escapist identities which have failed to produce wholeness and psychological well-being in the patient.

Our goal as clinicians is to facilitate the achievement of continuity within the self; that is, integration within the vertical axis of personality. A key element in this process is the resolution of ambivalence. In a sense, the situational somatizer, especially, has run out of options for failure. The split between mechanisms of defense/escape and the patient's existential problems has to be eliminated. If the patient can achieve this task, the outcome is positive and life-affirming; if s/he cannot do so, the possibility of personal growth and liberation will be frustrated if not altogether brought to a halt. This entire process depends on the ego-integrative defect. If it is mild to moderate, as in the case with the acute or situational somatizer, we tend to be optimistic about positive treatment outcomes. If the ego-integrative defect is severe, as has been noted in the case of chronic somatizers, we believe appropriate treatment involves a combination of psychopharmacology and therapeutic support in the forms of Cognitive-Behavioral and Dialectical Behavior Therapy, the goal being increased ego strength. We are inclined to believe a group identity is very helpful for these individuals, providing an atmosphere of acceptance and encouragement with the absence of psychological probing. To a certain extent, we understand much of the success in 12-step programs is due to the development of a group identity wherein persons can redefine themselves as empowered, sober, and healthy individuals. While it is unclear whether, or to what extent, this model may be effective in the treatment of somatization, the potential for somatizers to find a renewed capacity for functioning within the group context is significant.

Synesthenia, the mixing of sensory perceptions, is a rare and interesting phenomenon. As the reader is no doubt familiar, individuals with this condition may hear a word or number spoken and then see a color in response. A small portion of individuals possess developmental synesthesia and its manifestation appears in early childhood. Other individuals may experience this condition as the result of brain injury or sensory de-afferentation. There is also the possibility that synesthesia may result from the use of hallucinogenic drugs.[8] Although its etiology remains unclear, the phenomenon of synesthesia is intriguing because it exemplifies how sensory inputs can become confused and trigger atypical responses. The time may well come when we understand somatization in similar terms; that is, mistakes in neural processing resulting in bodily sensations displacing cognitive awareness. Certainly, Functional

MRI studies need to be carried out to evaluate the regions of the brain operative in both chronic and situational somatizers. The integration of the results of neuroscience with ego psychology will take us to the next level in our understanding of somatization.

The new buzzword in healthcare these days is "evidence-based." Everywhere you turn, you hear it. Pharmaceutical representatives tout their wares with the assurance that "evidence supports" one drug over another. Insurance case managers seem more likely to authorize payment for treatment that is "evidence-based." We've even used the phrase in the current volume, pointing out the benefits of utilizing objective testing in the diagnosis, treatment planning, and follow-up of somatizing patients. After years of relying, more or less, on individual clinical acumen, we health care professionals seem to be moving toward the opposite extreme. We want to know which treatments have demonstrated efficacy. One might say we want to hedge our bets. It makes a great deal of sense to try to situate our notions of effective treatment within the wider context of medical research. We are concerned for the welfare of our patients, mindful of the words we have sworn, first of all to do no harm. At the same time, we should not swing too far in the direction of reliance upon community opinion. Thinking outside the constraints of conventional wisdom may feel uncomfortable, but it has its place, and it's an important one. A case in point is Warren Warwick, former director of Cincinnati's Fairview-University Children's Hospital's cystic-fibrosis center for almost forty years.

> Warwick's combination of focus, aggressiveness, and inventiveness is what makes him extraordinary. He thinks hard about his patients, he pushes them, and he does not hesitate to improvise. Twenty years ago, while he was listening to a church choir and mulling over how he might examine his patients better, he came up with a new stethoscope—a stereo-stethoscope, he calls it. It has two bells dangling from it, and, because of a built-in sound delay, transmits lung sounds in stereo. He had an engineer make it for him. Listening to a patient with the instrument, he put one bell on the right side of her chest and the other on her left side, and insisted that he could systematically localize how individual lobes of her lungs sounded. He invented a new cough. It wasn't enough that his patients actively cough up their sputum. He wanted a deeper, better cough, and later, in his office, Warwick made another patient practice his cough. The patient stretched his arms upward, yawned, pinched his nose, bent down as far as he could, let the pressure build up, and then, straightening, blasted everything out. He produced his most far-reaching invention almost two decades ago—a mechanized, chest-thumping vest for patients to wear. Warwick's device was at least as effective as manual chest therapy, and was used far more consistently. Today, forty-five thousand patients with CF and other lung diseases use the technology.[9]

Warwick has described national clinical guidelines for care as "a record of the past, and little more—they should have an expiration date."[10]

If there is one theme that runs throughout the present volume, it is the authors' conviction that progress in the diagnosis and treatment of somatization will take place when clinicians take up the gauntlet of original thinking. We need to challenge our preconceptions and discard what no longer works, even if our community declares it as "evidence-based." Like the proverbial investment strategy, we do well not to place all of our eggs in one basket. But that is precisely what takes place when we attempt to fit our patients into one or another of typical DSM categories, ignoring the underlying pathology, and then wonder why they fail to get better. We need a renewed interest in personality theory and sensory perception with a view to more adequately conceptualizing the etiological factors in this patient population. As economics gain increasing importance in health care delivery, clinicians will find it necessary to evaluate psychosomatic populations with greater specificity and apply pharmacological and psychological interventions that have genuine potential for functional relief. The days of passing these patients from one clinician to another are coming to an end: The system simply can't afford it. For the clinician who is willing to think "outside the box" and consider new possibilities for diagnosis and treatment of conditions reflecting the mind-body interface, a challenging and fascinating future awaits.

Notes

INTRODUCTION

1. Katon, W. J. (no date) *Somatization and Primary Care*. http://courses.washington.edu/hubio516/Slides/Somatiz%20Prim%20Care.ppt.

2. Lin, E. H. (1991) Frustrating patients: physician and patient perspectives among distressed high users of medical services. *Journal of General Internal Medicine*, 6: 3, 241–46.

3. Fink, P. et al. (1999) Somatization in primary care: Prevalence, health care utilization, and general practitioner recognition. *Psychosomatics*, 40: 330–38.

CHAPTER 1

1. Barsky, A. J. (1983) Overview: Hypochondriasis, bodily complaints, and somatic styles. *American Journal of Psychiatry*, 140: 3, 273.

2. Hamlin, C., Hitchcock, M., Hoffmeister, J., & Owens, R. (1996) Predicting surgical outcome for pain relief and return to work. *Best Practice and Benchmarking in Healthcare*, 5: 258–61.

3. Barsky.

4. Webster, B. & Shook, S. (1994) The cost of compensable upper extremity cumulative trauma disorders. *Journal of Occupational Medicine,* 36: 7, 713–17.

5. Steckel, W. (1943) *The Interpretation of Dreams*. New York: Liveright; Lipowski, Z. Somatization: The concept and its clinical application. *American Journal of Psychiatry*, 145: 45, 358–68.

6. American Psychiatric Association. (2000) *Diagnostic and Statistical Manual of Mental Disorders IV-TR*. Washington, DC.

7. Lipowski; Barsky; Kellner, R. (1991) *Psychosomatic Syndromes and Somatic Symptoms*. Washington, DC: American Psychiatric Press, 189–226, 212–13.

8. Barksy, A. J. (1989) Somatoform disorders, in H. I. Kaplan and B. J. Saddock, eds. *Comprehensive Textbook of Psychiatry*, 5th ed. Baltimore: Williams & Wilkins, 1009–27.

9. Shorter, E. (1997) *A History of Psychiatry: From the Era of the Asylum to the Age of Prozac*. New York: John Wiley & Sons, Inc., 101.

10. Shorter, 106.

11. Shorter, 106.

12. Shorter, 107.

13. Malik, M. L. & Beutler, L. E. (2003) The emergence of dissatisfaction with the DSM, in L. Beutler & F. Malik (Eds.), *Redefining the DSM: A Psychological Perspective*. Washington, DC: American Psychological Association, 4.

14. Malik & Beutler, 6.

15. Malik & Beutler, 6.

16. Houts, A. C. (2003) Discovery, invention, and the expansion of the modern *Diagnostic and Statistical Manuals of Mental Disorders*, in L. Beutler & F. Malik (Eds.) *Redefining the DSM: A Psychological Perspective*. Washington, DC: American Psychological Association, 17–65.

17. Houts, 26–27

18. Houts, 27.

19. Houts, 39.

20. Houts, 39.

21. Houts, 40.

22. Houts, 41.

23. Houts, 47.

24. Houts, 47

25. Houts, 48.

26. Houts, 49.

27. Houts, 49.

28. Houts, 50.

29. Fauman, M. A. (1994) *Study Guide to DSM-IV*. Washington, DC: American Psychiatric Press, 5.

30. Malik & Beutler, 10.

31. Joiner, T. E. & Schmidt, N. B. (2003) Taxometrics can "do diagnostics right" (and it isn't quite as hard as you think), in L. Beutler & F. Malik (Eds.), *Redefining the DSM: A Psychological Perspective*. Washington, DC: American Psychological Association, 108.

32. Joiner & Schmidt, 109.

33. Joiner & Schmidt, 113.

34. Akiskal, H. S. (2004) The bipolar spectrum in psychiatric and general medical practice. *Primary Psychiatry*, 11: 9, 30.

35. Akiskal, 34.

36. Akiskal.

37. Tsuang, M. T. (2002) Schizotaxia and the prevention of schizophrenia, in J. E. Helzer & J. J. Hudziak (Eds.), *Defining Psychopathology in the 21st Century*. Washington, DC: American Psychiatric Publishing, Inc., 249–60.

38. Tsuang, 252.
39. Tsuang, 252.
40. Tsuang, 253.
41. Waddington, J. L, Scully, P. J., & O'Callaghan, E. (1997) "The new antipsychotics and their potential for early intervention in schizophrenia. *Schizophrenia Research*, 28: 2–3, 207–22.
42. Tsuang, 258.
43. American Psychiatric Association. (2000) *Diagnostic and Statistical Manual of Mental Disorders IV-TR*, Washington, DC, Author, 485.
44. DSM-IV-TR, 485.
45. Fauman, 246.
46. DSM-IV-TR, 490.
47. Fauman, 246.
48. DSM-IV-TR, 490.
49. DSM-IV-TR, 486.
50. DSM-IV-TR, 486.
51. Rief, W. & Hiller, W. (1999) Toward empirically based criteria for the classification of somatoform disorders. *Journal of Psychosomatic Research*, 46: 6, 507.
52. DSM-IV-TR, 492.
53. DSM-IV-TR, 511
54. Fauman, 9.
55. Escobar, J. I., Swartz, M., Rubio-Stipec, M., & Manu, P. (1991) Medically unexplained symptoms: Distribution, risk factors, and comorbidity, in Lawrence J. Kirmayer & James M. Robbins (Eds.), *Current Concepts of Somatization: Research and Clinical Perspectives*, Washington, DC: American Psychiatric Press, Inc., 67.
56. Escobar et al., 67.
57. Escobar et al., 67.
58. Allen, L. A. et al. (2001) Somatization: A delibitating syndrome in primary care. *Psychosomatics*, 42: 63–67, 63.
59. Allen et al., 63, 65.
60. Robbins, J. M. & Kirmayer, L. J. (1991) Cognitive and social factors in somatization, in Lawrence J. Kirmayer & James M. Robbins (Eds.), *Current Concepts of Somatization: Research and Clinical Perspectives*. Washington, DC: American Psychiatric Press, Inc., 107.
61. Robbins & Kirmayer, 108.
62. Robbins & Kirmayer, 114.
63. Robbins & Kirmayer, 125.
64. Robbins & Kirmayer, 108; Leibbrand, R. & Hiller. (2000) Hypochondriasis and somatization: Two distinct aspects of somatoform disorders. *Journal of Clinical Psychology*, 56: 1, 63–72.
65. Barsky, A. J., Wyshak, G., & Klerman, G. L. (1992) Psychiatric comorbidity in DSM-III-R hypochondriasis. *Archives of General Psychiatry*, 49: 2, 101–8.
66. Robbins & Kirmayer, 125.
67. (No Author) (2004) Depression and physical symptoms: The mind-body connection. *Journal of Clinical Psychiatry*, 65: 6, 867–76.

68. Martin, R. D. (1999) The somatoform conundrum: A question of nosological values. *General Hospital Psychiatry*, 21: 178.
69. Martin, 178.
70. Martin, 178.
71. Martin, 178.
72. Martin, 179.
73. Martin, 184.
74. Martin, 184.
75. Martin, 184.
76. Martin, 184.
77. Sharpe, M. & Carson, A. (2001) "Unexplained" somatic symptoms, functional syndromes, and somatization: Do we need a paradigm shift? *Annals of Internal Medicine*, 134: 926.
78. Sharpe & Carson, 926.
79. Sharpe & Carson, 926.
80. Sharpe & Carson, 927.
81. Sharpe & Carson, 927.
82. Sharpe & Carson, 929.
83. Sharpe & Carson, 929.

CHAPTER 2

1. Barsky, A. J. (1983) Overview: Hypochondriasis, bodily complaints, and somatic styles. *American Journal of Psychiatry*, 140: 3, 273.
2. Barsky, 273.
3. Hamlin, C., Hitchcock, M., Hoffmeister, J., & Owens, R. (1996) Predicting surgical outcome for pain relief and return to work. *Best Practice and Benchmarking in Healthcare*, 5: 258–61.
4. Hamlin et al.
5. Bass, C. & Murphy, M. (1995) Somatoform and personality disorders: Syndromal comorbidity and overlapping developmental pathways. *Journal of Psychosomatic Research*, 39: 403; Smith, W. L., Hamlin, C., & Jonassen, E. A. (1999) Somatization: An independent variable influencing surgical outcome for pain relief. *Oakleaf,* USN MSC.
6. Stahl, S. (2000) Blue genes and the mechanism of action of antidepressants. *Journal of Clinical Psychiatry*, 6l: 3, 164–65.
7. Hollander, E. (1993) *Obsessive-Compulsive Disorders.* Washington, DC: American Psychiatric Press.
8. Hollander.
9. Hellman, K. M., Barrett, A. M., & Adair, J. C. (1998) Possible mechanisms of anosognosia: A defect in self-awareness. *Philosophical Transactions of the Royal Society of London, Series B, Biological Sciences*, 353: 1377, 1903–909.
10. Pia, L. & Tamietto, M. (2006) Unawareness in schizophrenia: Neuropsychological and neuroanatomical findings. *Psychiatry and Clinical Neurosciences*,

60: 5, 531–37.

11. Edwards, R. R., Doleys, D. M., Fillingim, R. B., & Lowery, D. (2001) Ethnic differences in pain tolerance: Clinical implications in a chronic pain population. *Psychosomatic Medicine*, 63: 2, 316–23.

12. Bachiocco, V., Scesi, M., Morselli, A. M., & Carli, G. (1993) Individual pain history and familial pain tolerance models: Relationships to post-surgical pain. *The Clinical Journal of Pain*, 9: 4, 266–71.

13. Bragdon et al.

14. de Wied, M. & Verbaten, D. M. (2001) Affective pictures processing, attention, and pain tolerance. *Pain*, 90: 1–2, 163–72.

15. de Wied & Verbaten.

CHAPTER 3

1. Corey, G. (1991) *Theory and Practice of Counseling and Psychotherapy*. Pacific Grove: Brooks/Cole Publishing Company, 213.

2. Rief, W. (2007) Analyzing the problems managing patients with medically unexplained symptoms. *Journal of General Internal Medicine*, 22: 5, 704–6; Lynch, D. J. et al. (2007) The patient-physician relationship and medical utilization. *The Primary Care Companion to the Journal of Clinical Psychiatry*, 9: 4, 266–70.

3. Halpern, J. (2007) Empathy and patient-physician conflicts. *Journal of General Internal Medicine*, 22: 5, 697.

4. Descartes, R. (1981) Discourse on the method. In E. S. Haldane & G. R. T. Ross (Trans.), *The Philosophical Works of Descartes* (Vol. 1). Cambridge: Cambridge University Press, 101.

5. Descartes, 101.

6. Levi, A. F. (1959) *Philosophy and the Modern World*. Bloomington: Indiana University Press, 33.

7. Renik, O. (1993) Analytic interaction: Conceptualizing technique in light of the analyst's irreducible subjectivity. *Psychoanalytic Quarterly*, 62: 553–71; Ogden, T. H. (1994). The analytic third: working with intersubjective clinical facts. *International Journal of Psychoanalysis*, 75: 3–19.

8. Gabbard, G. O. (1996) A reconsideration of objectivity in the analyst. *International Journal of Psychoanalysis*, 78: 15–26.

9. Gabbard, 15.

10. Gabbard, 10.

11. Gabbard, 10.

12. Brown, W. A. (1998). The placebo effect. *Scientific American*, 278: 90–95.

13. Brown, W. A., Johnson, M. F., & Chen, Mon-Gy (1992). Clinical features of depressed patients who do and do not improve with placebo. *Psychiatry Research*, 41: 203–14.

14. Brown, Johnson, & Chen.

15. Frank, J. (1961). *Persuasion and Healing*. Baltimore: The Johns Hopkins University Press.

16. Brown, W. A. (2002). Are antidepressants as ineffective as they look? *Prevention and Treatment*, 5, Article 25.

17. Mayberg, H. S. et al. (2002) The functional neuroanatomy of the placebo effect. *American Journal of Psychiatry*, 159: 728–37.

18. Mayberg et al.

19. Gabbard, G. O. (2000). A neurobiologically informed perspective on psychotherapy. *The British Journal of Psychiatry*, 177: 117–22.

20. Liggan, D. Y. & Kay, J. (2005) Some neurobiological aspects of psychotherapy: A review. In Taming the anxious mind: How psychotherapy and medications transform the brain, CME. Cochairs: Philip T. Ninan, MD; Michael R. Liebowitz, MD; Faculty: Boadie W. Dunlop, MD; Sarah A. Feigon, PhD; Reviewer: Daniel K. Winstead, MD, www.medscape.com.

21. Johansson, B. B. (2004) Brain plasticity in health and disease. *Keio Journal of Medicine,* 53: 4, 231.

22. Johansson, 231.

23. Schuessler, G. (2003) Neurobiology and psychotherapy. Lecture given at the Congress in Innsbruck on "Neurobiology and Psychotherapy." www.v-r.de/data/files/117219/schuessler.pdf, 1–24.

24. Johansson, 234.

25. Schwartz J., Stoessel P, Baxter L., et al. (1996) Systematic changes in cerebral glucose metabolic rate after successful behavior modification treatment of obsessive compulsive behavior. *Archives of General Psychiatry*, 53: 109–13.

26. Knowlton, L. (2001) PET scans compare effects of drug treatment and talk therapy. *Psychiatric Times*, 18: 7. http://psychiatrictimes.com/p010744.html.

27. Brody et al.

28. Paquette, V. et al. (2003) "Change the mind and you change the brain": Effects of cognitive-behavior therapy on the neural correlates of spider phobia. *NeuroImage* 18, article in press, 1–9.

29. Paquette.

30. Roffman, J. (2005) Neuroimaging and the functional neuroanatomy of psychotherapy. *Psychological Medicine*, 28: 1–14.

31. Liggan & Kay, no page number.

32. Liggan & Kay, no page number.

CHAPTER 4

1. Stein, M. (1983) *In Midlife: A Jungian Perspective*. Dallas: Spring Publications, Inc.

2. Albertson, B., Brehm, J. R., & Alvarez, M. Ambivalence as experienced conflict. January 1, 2004. http://cas.uchicago.edu/workshops/polpsych/ambivalence.pdf.

3. Saddock, B. J. and Saddock, V. A. (2000) Typical signs and symptoms of psychiatric illness, in Benjamin J. Saddock & Virginia A. Saddock (Eds.), *Comprehensive Textbook of Psychiatry*, 7th ed., Baltimore: Williams & Wilkins, 678.

4. Chayes, M. F. (1989) Concerning certain vicissitudes of denial in personality development, in E. L. Edelstein, Donald L. Nathanson, & Andrew M. Stone (Eds.), *Denial: A Clarification of Concepts and Research*. New York: Plenum Press, 100.
5. Ostow, M. (1968) The consequences of ambivalence. *Psychosomatics*, 9: 257–58.
6. Ostow, 256.
7. Ostow, 258.
8. John Philip Smith, letter to author, 10 October 2004.
9. John 15:13 KJV.
10. John Philip Smith, letter to author, 10 October 2004.
11. Chayes, 99.
12. Marty, P. (1968) A major process of somatization: The progressive disorganization. *International Journal of Psychoanalysis*, 49: 2, 246–49.
13. Marty, 247.
14. Leary, T. (1957) *The Interpersonal Diagnosis of Personality*. New York: The Ronald Press Co.
15. Marty, 247.
16. Rodin, G. M. (1984) Somatization and the self: Psychotherapeutic issues. *American Journal of Psychotherapy*, 38: 2, 257–63.
17. Rodin, 258.
18. Shakespeare, W. *The Tragedy of Hamlet: The Prince of Denmark*. Act III, Scene I. Project Gutenberg, Champagne, IL, 22.
19. Peterson. C. (1987) To be or not to be: A study of ambivalence. *Journal of Analytical Psychology*, 81.
20. Peterson, 81.

CHAPTER 5

1. Singer, T. et al. (2004) Empathy for pain involves the affective but not sensory components of pain. *Science*, 303: 1157–162.
2. Singer.
3. Singer.
4. Wolff, W. (1950) *Values and Personality: An Existential Psychology of Crisis*. New York: Grune & Stratton, 18.
5. Wolff, 19.
6. Sullivan, H. S. (1954) *The Psychiatric Interview*. New York: W.W. Norton & Company, 207.
7. Nathanson, D. L. (1996) About emotion, in Donald L. Nathanson (Ed.) *Knowing Feeling: Affect, Script, and Psychotherapy*. New York: W. W. Norton & Company, 3.
8. Wolff, 18–19.
9. Wolff, 19.
10. Wolff, 21–22.
11. Wolff, 23.
12. Wolff, 23.

13. Wolff, 23.
14. Wolff, 23.
15. Glass, J. M. (2008) Fibromyalgia and cognition, in Laurence A. Bradley, Lesley M. Arnold, Jennifer M. Glass, & Daniel J. Clauw, Understanding fibromyalgia and its related disorders, *Primary Care Companion, Journal of Clinical Psychiatry*, 10: 2, 137.
16. Leary, T. (1957). *The Interpersonal Diagnosis of Personality*. New York: The Ronald Press Co.

CHAPTER 6

1. Hakula et al.
2. Tumlin, T. R. (2001). Treating chronic-pain patients in psychotherapy. *Journal of Clinical Psychology*, 57: 11, 1276.
3. Kooiman, C. G. et al. (2003). Is alexithymia a risk factor for unexplained physical symptoms in general medical outpatients? *Psychosomatic Medicine*, 65: 911–18.
4. Porcelli, P. et al. (1992). Alexithymia as predictor of treatment outcome in patients with functional gastrointestinal disorders. *Journal of Psychosomatic Research*, 36, 5: 417–24.
5. Taylor, G. J., Parker, J. D., Bagby, R. M., & Acklin, M. W. (1997). Alexithymia and somatic complaints in psychiatric out-patients. *Comprehensive Psychiatry*, 38: 3, 160–65.
6. Blaustein, J. P. & Tuber, S. B. (1998) Knowing the unspeakable: Somatization as an expression of disruptions in affective-relational functioning. *Bulletin of the Menninger Clinic*, 62: 3, 355.
7. Smith, W. L. (1967) A psychotherapeutic technique for resolving impasse resistance. *Psychotherapy: Theory, Research, & Practice*, 4: 162–63.
8. Leary, T. (1957) *The Interpersonal Diagnosis of Personality*. New York: The Ronald Press Co., 360–61, 402.
9. Leary, 246.
10. Leary, 246.
11. Leary, 247.
12. Leary, 247.
13. Leary, 303.
14. Leary, 323.
15. Cloninger, C. R., Reich, T., & Guze, G. B. (1975) A multifactorial model of disease transmission: Familial relationships between sociopaths and hysteria. *British Journal of Psychiatry*, 127: 23–32.
16. Price, J. S., Gardner Jr., R., & Erickson, M. (2004) Can depression, anxiety and somatization be understood as appeasement displays? *Journal of Affective Disorders*, 79: 5.
17. Price, Gardner, & Erickson, 6.
18. Leary, 293.

19. Leary, 315.
20. Leary, 402.
21. Leary, 294–95.
22. Leary, 304.
23. Leary, 304.
24. Leary.
25. Kopp, R. & Kivel, C. (1990) Traps and escapes: An Adlerian approach to understanding resistance and resolving impasses in psychotherapy. *Individual Psychology*, 46: 2, 140.
26. Kopp & Kivel, 140–41.
27. Adler.

CHAPTER 7

1. Guthrie, E. (1991) Brief psychotherapy with patients with refractory irritable bowel syndrome. *British Journal of Psychotherapy*, 8: 175–88.
2. Kroenke, K. & Swindle, R. (2000) Cognitive-behavioral therapy for somatization and symptom syndromes: A critical review of controlled clinical trials. *Psychotherapy and Psychosomatics*, 69: 4, 205–15; Looper, K. J. & Kirmayer, L. J. (2002) Behavioral medicine approaches to somatoform disorders. *Journal of Consulting and Clinical Psychology*, 70: 3, 810–27; Hickie, I. B., Scott, E. M., & Davenport, T. A. (1998) Somatic distress: Developing more integrated concepts. *Current Opinion in Psychiatry*, 11: 2, 153–58.
3. Turk, D. C., Meichenbaum, D., & Genest, M. (1983) *Pain and Behavioral Medicine: A Cognitive-Behavioral Perspective*. New York: The Guilford Press, 4.
4. Turk, Meichenbaum, & Genest, 4.
5. Turk, Meichenbaum, & Genest, 4–5.
6. Beck, A. T., Rush, A. J., Shaw, B. F., & Emery, G. (1979) *Cognitive Theory of Depression*. New York: Guilford; Beck, A. T. (1976) *Cognitive Therapy and the Emotional Disorders*. New York: International Universities Press.
7. Rush, J. & Beck, A. T. (2000) Cognitive therapy, in Benjamin J. Saddock & Virginia A. Saddock (Eds.) *Comprehensive Textbook of Psychiatry*, 7th ed. Philadelphia: Lippincott Williams & Wilkins, 2167.
8. Neenan, M. & Dryden, M. (2004) *Cognitive Therapy: 100 Key Points and Techniques*. Hove & New York: Brunner-Routledge, 15.
9. Keenan & Dryden, 203.
10. Beck, A. T., Rush, J. A., Shaw, B. F., & Emery, G. (1979) *Cognitive Theory of Depression*. New York: The Guilford Press, 12–13.
11. Beck et al., 13.
12. Rush & Beck, 2170.
13. Friedman, E. S., Thase, M. E., & Wright, J. H. (2003) Cognitive and behavioral therapies, in Allan Tasman, Jerald Kay, & Jeffrey A. Lieberman (Eds.) *Psychiatry: Therapeutics*, 2nd ed. Chichester, England: John Wiley & Sons, Ltd., 56.
14. Friedman, Thase, & Wright, 57.

15. Rush & Beck, 2170.

16. Sharpe, M. (1995) Cognitive behavioural therapies in the treatment of functional somatic symptoms, in R. Mayou, C. Bass, & M. Sharpe (Eds.) New York: Oxford University Press, 124, 126.

17. Sharpe, 126.

18. Taerk, G. (1998) Psychotherapy of functional somatic syndromes, in Peter Manu (Ed.), *Functional Somatic Syndromes*. London: Cambridge University Press, 239.

19. Salkovskis, P. M. (1989) Somatic problems, in K. Hawton, P. M. Salkovskis, J. Kirk, & D. M. Clark, *Cognitive Behavioral Therapy for Psychiatric Problems: A Practical Guide*. Oxford: Oxford University Press, 241.

20. Salkovskis, 241.

21. Robbins, J. M. & Kirmayer, L. J. (1991) Cognitive and social factors in somatization, in Lawrence J. Kirmayer & James M. Robbins (Eds.), *Current Concepts of Somatization: Research and Clinical Perspectives*. Washington, DC: American Psychiatric Press, Inc., 113.

22. Taerk, 241.

23. Meichenbaum, D. (1993) Changing conceptions of cognitive behavior modification: Retrospect and prospect. *Journal of Consulting and Clinical Psychology*, 61: 2, 202.

24. Meichenbaum (1993), 203.

25. Meichenbaum (1993), 203.

26. Hoyt, M. F. & Meichenbaum, D. (1994) A conversation with Donald Meichenbaum. www.behavior.net/column/meichenbaum, 2.

27. Hoyt & Meichenbaum, 2.

28. Meichenbaum (1993), 203.

29. Hoyt & Meichenbaum, 3.

30. Hoyt & Meichenbaum, 3.

31. Hoyt & Meichenbaum, 6.

32. Hoyt & Meichenbaum, 5.

33. Meichenbaum (1993), 203.

34. Hoyt & Meichenbaum, 6.

36. Meichenbaum (1993), 204.

37. Meichenbaum (1993), 204.

38. Meichenbaum (1994), 9.

39. Meichenbaum (1994), 10.

40. Meichenbaum, D. (1977) *Cognitive-Behavior Modification: An Integrative Approach*. New York: Plenum Press, 148–49.

41. Meichenbaum (1977), 149.

42. Meichenbaum, D. (1996) Stress inoculation training for coping with stressors, *The Clinical Psychologist*, 49: 4–7.

43. Meichenbaum, D. (1996), 4.

44. Meichenbaum, D. (1996), 4.

45. Meichenbaum, D. (1996), 4.

46. Meichenbaum, D. (1996), 5.

47. Meichenbaum, D. (1996), 5; Meichenbaum, D. (1976) Cognitive factors in

biofeedback therapy. *Biofeedback and Self Regulation*, 1: 2, 201–16.

48. Meichenbaum (1976), 203.
49. Meichenbaum (1976), 203–4.
50. Meichenbaum (1976), 205.
51. Meichenbaum (1976), 206.
52. Meichenbaum (1976), 208–9.
53. Meichenbaum (1977), 170–71.
54. Meichenbaum (1977), 174.
55. Meichenbaum (1977), 174–75.
56. Meichenbaum (1977), 175.
57. Meichenbaum (1977), 175–76.
58. Fowler, J. W. & Keen, S. (1985) *Life-Maps: Conversations on the Journey of Faith*. Waco, TX: Word, Inc., 34.
59. Fowler & Keen, 34.
60. Fowler & Keen, 34.

CHAPTER 8

1. Linehan, M. M. (1993a) *Cognitive-Behavioral Treatment of Borderline Personality Disorder*. New York: The Guilford Press.
2. Evans, K. et al. (1999) Manual-assisted cognitive-behavioral therapy (MCAT): A randomized controlled trial of a brief intervention with bibliotherapy in the treatment of recurrent deliberate self-harm. *Psychological Medicine*, 29, 1–25; Wiser, S. & Telch, C. F. (1999) DBT for binge-eating disorder. *Journal of Clinical Psychology*, 55, 755–68; Linehan, M. M. et al. (1999) Dialectical behavior therapy for patients with borderline personality disorder and drug dependence. *American Journal on Addictions*, 8, 279–92.
3. Porter Adventist Hospital, Department of Psychiatry, 2525 S. Downing St., Denver, CO, 80210.
4. Bass, C. & Murphy, M. (1995) Somatoform and personality disorders: Syndromal comorbidity and overlapping developmental pathways. *Journal of Psychosomatic Research*, 39: 403; Sansone, R. A. & Sansone, L. A. (2003) Borderline personality: Different symptoms in different treatment settings? *International Journal of Psychiatry in Clinical Practice*, 7: 3, 187–91.
5. Stuart, S. & Noyes, R. (1999) Attachment and interpersonal communication in somatization. *Psychosomatics*, 40: 34–43.
6. Linehan (1993a), 47.
7. Linehan (1993a), 49.
8. Linehan (1993a), 50.
9. Linehan (1993a), 51.
10. Linehan (1993a), 51.
11. Linehan (1993a), 51.
12. Linehan (1993a), 51.
13. Linehan (1993a), 10–11.

14. Linehan (1993a), 11.
15. Linehan (1993a), 11.
16. Linehan (1993a), 11.
17. Linehan (1993a), 221.
18. Linehan (1993a), 221.
19. (No Author) (2003) *Dialectical Behavior Therapy Intensive Training Course (Manual)*. Seattle, WA: Behavioral Tech, LLC, 32.
20. *Manual*, 65.
21. *Manual*, 65.
22. *Manual*, 65.
23. *Manual*, 66.
24. Linehan (1993a), 302.
25. *Manual*, 66.
26. Linehan (1993a), 338–39.
27. *Manual*, 71.
28. Linehan (1993a), 144.
29. *Manual*, 107.
30. Linehan (1993a), 107.
31. Linehan, M. M. (1993b) *Skills Training Manual for Treating Borderline Personality Disorder*. New York: The Guilford Press, 167–69.
32. Linehan (1993b), 170–73.
33. Linehan (1993a), 149.
34. Linehan (1993a), 149.
35. Linehan (1993a), 149.
36. Linehan (1993a), 149
37. Nathanson, D. L. (1996) About emotion, in Donald L. Nathanson (Ed.) *Knowing Feeling: Affect, Script, and Psychotherapy*. New York: W. W. Norton & Company, 3.
38. Linehan (1993a), 149.
39. Linehan (1993a), 149.
40. Linehan (1993b), 254.
41. Linehan (1993a), 150.
42. Linehan (1993a), 150.
43. Linehan (1993a), 152.
44. Linehan (1993a), 20.
45. Linehan (1993a), 20.
46. Linehan (1993a), 21.
47. *Manual*, 32.
48. Linehan (1993a), 373.
49. Linehan (1993a), 374.
50. Linehan (1993a), 21.
51. Linehan (1993a), 21.
52. Hegel, G. W. F. (1952) *Hegel's Phenomenology of Spirit*, A. V. Miller (Trans.) Oxford: Oxford University Press; Marx, K. & Engels, F. (1970) *Selected Works* (Vol. III). New York: International.
53. Linehan (1993a), 34.

54. Wienfried, R. & Barsky, A. J. (2005) Psychobiological perspectives on somatoform disorders. *Psychoneuroendocrinology*, 30: 10, 996–1002.
55. Stuart, S. & Noyes, R., 1.
56. Stuart, S. & Noyes, R., 1.
57. Linehan (1993a), 80.
58. Linehan (1993a), 81.
59. Linehan (1993a), 213.

CHAPTER 9

1. Strasser, F. & Strasser. A. (1997) *Existential Time-Limited Therapy: The Wheel of Existence*. New York: John Wiley & Sons, 16–19.
2. Levi, A. F. (1959) *Philosophy and the Modern World*. Bloomington: Indiana University Press.
3. Wolff, W. (1950) *Values and Personality: An Existential Psychology of Crisis*. New York: Grune & Stratton, x.
4. Wolff, 5.
5. Van Deurzen, E. (1998) *Paradox and Passion in Psychotherapy: An Existential Approach to Therapy and Counseling*. New York: John Wiley & Sons, 144.
6. Yalom, I. (1980) *Existential Psychotherapy*. New York: Basic Books, 9.
7. Vaillant, G. E. (1993) *The Wisdom of the Ego*. Cambridge, MA: Harvard University Press.
8. Yalom, I. (2002) *The Gift of Therapy*. New York: Harper Collins Publishers, 43.
9. Tillich, P. (1957) *Dynamics of Faith*. New York: Harper & Row, Publishers, 42.
10. Wolff, 21.
11. Schreurs, A. (2002) *Psychotherapy and Spirituality: Integrating the Spiritual Dimension into Therapeutic Practice*. London: Jessica Kingsley Publishers, 138.
12. Yalom (2002), xiv.
13. Yalom (2002), 5.
14. Yalom, I. (1980), 8–9.
15. Yalom (2002), xiii–xiv.
16. Strasser & Strasser, 18.
17. Strasser & Strasser, 18.
18. Strasser & Strasser, 18.
19. Strasser & Strasser, 53.
20. Strasser & Strasser, 53.
21. Keshen, A. (2006) A new look at existential psychotherapy. *American Journal of Psychotherapy*, 60: 3, 292.
22. Keshen, 292–93.
23. Carlat, D. J. (1998) The psychiatric review of symptoms: A screening tool for family physicians, *The American Family Physician*, 58: 7, 1668–671.

24. Freud, S. ([1924] 1958) The dynamics of transference, in J. Strachey (Ed. and Trans.), *The Complete Psychological Works of Sigmund Freud* (Vol. 12, 99–108). London: The Hogarth Press.

25. Sedgewick, D. (1994) *The Wounded Healer: Countertransference from a Jungian Perspective*. London: Routledge; Little, M. (1981) Counter-transference and the patient's response to it, in R. Langs (Ed.), *Classics in Psychoanalytic Technique* (143–51). New York: Jason Aronson.

26. Little, 145.

CHAPTER 10

1. Han, C. et al. (2008) Fluoxetine versus sertraline in the treatment of patients with undifferentiated somatoform disorder: A randomized, open-label, 12-week, parallel-group trial. *Progress in Neuropsychopharmacology and Biological Psychiatry*, 32: 2, 437–44.

2. O'Malley, P. G. et al. (1999) Antidepressant therapy for unexplained symptoms and symptom syndromes. *Journal of Family Practice*. 48: 12, 980–90.

3. Smith, G. G. et al. (2000) Consultation-liaison psychiatrist's management of somatoform disorders. *Psychosomatics*. 41, 481–89.

4. Fallon, B. A. et al. (2008) A double-masked, placebo-controlled study of fluoxetine for hypochondriasis. *Journal of Clinical Psychopharmacology*. 28: 6, 638–45.

5. Phillips, K. A. (2002) A randomized, placebo-controlled trial of fluoxetine in body dysmorphic disorder. *Archives of General Psychiatry*. 59: 4, 381–88.

6. Harth, W. et al. (2007) Psychopharmacological treatment of dermatological patients—when simply talking does not help. *Journal der Deutschen Dermatologischen Gesellschaft*, 5: 12, 1101–6.

7. Denninger, J. W. et al. (2006) Somatic symptoms in outpatients with major depressive disorder treated with fluoxetine. *Psychosomatics*. 47: 4, 348–52.

8. Voznesenskaia, T. G. (1999) Prozac treatment of chronic tension headache, *Zhurnal Nevrologii i Psikhiatrii Imeni S.S. Korsakova*. 99: 1, 34–36.

9. Han, 2008.

10. Denninger, 2006.

11. Hoss, D. & Segal, S. (1998) Scalp dysesthesia. *Archives of Dermatology*, 134: 3, 327–30.

12. Staab, J. P, Ruckenstein, M. J., & Amsterdam, J. D. (2004) A prospective trial of sertraline for chronic subjective dizziness. *Laryngoscope*, 114: 9, 1637–641.

13. Alpay, F. B. & Turhan, N. O. (2001) Intermittent versus continuous sertraline therapy in the treatment of premenstrual dysphoric disorders. *International Journal of Fertility and Women's Medicine*, 46: 4, 228–31.

14. Okugawa, G. (2002) Paroxetine for treatment of somatization disorder. *Journal of Neuropsychiatry and Clinical Neurosciences*, 14, 464–65.

15. Creed, F. (2008) The relationship between somatization and outcome in patients with severe irritable bowel syndrome. *Journal of Psychosomatic Research*, 64: 6, 613–20.

16. Doraiswamy, P. M. (2006) A randomized controlled trial of paroxetine for noncardiac chest pain. *Psychopharmacology Bulletin*, 29: 1, 15–24.

17. Voon, V. & Lang, A. E. (2005) Antidepressant treatment outcomes of psychogenic movement disorder. *Journal of Clinical Psychiatry*, 66: 12, 1529–534.

18. Croom, K. F., Perry, C. M., & Plosker, G. L. (2009) Mirtazapine: A review of its use in major depression and other psychiatric disorders, *CNS Drugs*, 23: 5, 427–52.

19. Han, C. et al. (2008) Venlafaxine versus mirtazapine in the treatment of undifferentiated somatoform disorder: A 12-week prospective, open-label, randomized, parallel-group trial. *Clinical Drug Investigation*, 28: 4, 251–61; Menza, M. et al. (2001) Treatment of somatization disorder with nefazodone: A prospective, open-label study. *Annals of Clinical Psychiatry*, 13: 3, 1040–297.

20. Kjernisted, K., Enns, M. W., & Lander, M. (2002) An open-label clinical trial of nefazedone in hypochondriasis. *The Academy of Psychosomatic Medicine*, 43, 290–94.

21. Muller, J. E. et al. (2008) Escitalopram in the treatment of multisomatoform disorder: a double-blind, placebo controlled trial. *International Clinical Psychopharmacology*, 23: 1, 43–48.

22. Muller.

23. Aragona, M. et al. (2005) Randomized double-blind comparison of serotonergic (citalopram) versus noradrenergic (reboxetine) reuptake inhibitors in outpatients with somatoform, DSM-IV-TR pain disorder. *European Journal of Pain*, 9: 1, 33–38.

24. Volz, H. P. et al. (2002) St. John's wort extract (LI 160) in somatoform disorders: Results of a placebo-controlled trial. *Psychopharmacology (Berlin)*, 164: 3, 294–300.

25. Volz, 2002.

26. Volz, 2002.

27. Keeley, R., Smith, M., & Miller, J. (2000) Somatoform symptoms and treatment nonadherence in depressed family medicine outpatients. *Archives of Family Medicine*, 9: 46–54.

28. O'Malley, 1999.

29. Hurwitz, T. A. (2003) Somatization and Conversion Disorder. *Canadian Journal of Psychiatry*, 49: 172–78.

30. Greco, T., Eckert, G., & Kroenke, K. (2004) The outcome of physical symptoms with treatment of depression. *Journal of General Internal Medicine*, 18: 8, 813–18.

31. Goldstein, D. J. et al. (2004) Effects of duloxetine on painful physical symptoms associated with depression. *Psychosomatics*, 45: 17–28.

32. Spielmans, G. I. (2008) Duloxetine does not relieve painful physical symptoms in depression: A meta-analysis. *Psychotherapy and Psychosomatics*, 77: 1, 12–16.

33. Humberto, M. & Escobar, J. I. (2008) Unexplained physical symptoms: What's a psychiatrist to do? *Psychiatric Times*, 25: 9, Special Report.

34. Henningsen, P. & Lowe, B. (2006) Depression, pain, and somatoform disorders. *Current Opinion in Psychiatry*, 19: 1, 19–24.

35. Sayar, K., Barsky, A. J., & Gulec, H. (2005) Does somatosensory amplification decrease with antidepressant treatment? *The Academy of Psychosomatic Medicine*, 46: 340–44.

36. Hand, M. (1999) Antidepressant treatment of patients with diffuse esophageal spasm: A psychosomatic approach. *Journal of Clinical Gastroenterology*, 28: 3, 228–32.

37. Maurer, I., Volz, H. P., & Sauer, H. (1999) Gabapentin leads to remission of somatoform pain disorder with major depression. *Pharmacopsychiatry*, 32: 6, 255–57.

38. Garcia-Campayo, J. & Sanz-Carillo, C. (2001) Gabapentin for the treatment of patients with somatization disorder. *Journal of Clinical Psychiatry*, 62: 6, 474.

39. Stahl, S. M. (2004) Anticonvulsants and the relief of chronic pain: Pregabalin and gabapentin as $\alpha_w\delta$ ligands at voltage-gated calcium channels. *Journal of Clinical Psychiatry*, 65: 5, 596–97.

40. Stahl, 597.

41. Stahl.

42. Chand, P. K., Anand, S., & Murthy, P. (2000) A case of monosymptomatic hypochondriacal psychosis treated with olanzapine. *Annals of Clinical Psychiatry*, 12: 4, 247–49.

43. Mercan, S. et al. (2007) Atypical antipsychotic drugs in the treatment of delusional parasitosis. *International Journal of Psychiatry and Medicine*, 47: 1, 29–37.

44. Personal communication.

45. Schatzberg, A. F., Cole, J. O., & DeBattista, C. (2007) *Manual of Clincal Psychopharmacology*. Washington, DC: American Psychiatric Press, 469.

46. Zorumski, C. F., Rubin, E. H., & Burke, W. J. (1988) Electroconvulsive therapy for the elderly: A review. *Hospital and Community Psychiatry*, 39: 6, 643–47.

47. Zorumski et al.

48. Rasmussen, K. G. et al. (2004) Relationship between somatization and remission with ECT. *Psychiatry Research*, 129: 3, 293–95.

49. Newmark, T. S. & Al-Samarrai, S. (2004) Hypochondriasis and ECT. *Psychosomatics*, 45: 1, 90–91; Daniel, W. F., Yeo, R. A., & Smith, J. E. (1989) Conversion disorders and ECT. *British Journal of Psychiatry*, 154, 274–75.

50. Fink, M. (2007) Complaints of loss of personal memories after electroconvulsive therapy: evidence of a somatoform disorder? *Psychosomatics*, 48: 4, 290–93.

CHAPTER 11

1. Wolff, W. (1950) *Values and Personality: An Existential Psychology of Crisis*. New York: Grune & Stratton, 50.

2. Wolff, 50.

3. Wolff, 50.

4. Wolff, 50.

5. Wolff, 50.

6. Vaillant, G. E. (1993) *The Wisdom of the Ego*. Cambridge, MA: Harvard University Press, 240.

7. Vaillant, 240.

8. Grossenbacher, P. G. & Lovelace, C. T. (2001) Mechanisms of synesthesia: Cognitive and physiological constraints. *Trends in Cognitive Sciences*, 5: 1, 36–41.

9. Gawande, A. The Bell Curve, in *The New Yorker*, December 6, 2004.

10. Warwick.

Bibliography

BOOKS AND ARTICLES IN BOOKS

American Psychiatric Association. (2000) *Diagnostic and Statistical Manual of Mental Disorders: IV-TR*. Washington, DC.

Barksy, A. J. (1989) Somatoform disorders, in Kaplan, H. I. & Saddock, B. J. (Eds.) *Comprehensive Textbook of Psychiatry*, 5th ed. Baltimore: Williams & Wilkins, 1009–27.

Beck, A. T., Rush, J. A., Shaw, B. F., & Emery, G. (1979) *Cognitive Theory of Depression*. New York: The Guilford Press.

Beck, A. T. (1976) *Cognitive Therapy and the Emotional Disorders*. New York: International Universities Press.

Chayes, M. F. (1989) Concerning certain vicissitudes of denial in personality development, in E. L. Edelstein, Donald L. Nathanson, & Andrew M. Stone (Eds.), *Denial: A Clarification of Concepts and Research*, New York: Plenum Press.

Corey, G. (1991) *Theory and Practice of Counseling and Psychotherapy*. Pacific Grove, CA: Brooks/Cole Publishing Company.

Descartes, R. (1981) Discourse on the Method, in E. S. Haldane & G. R. T. Ross (Trans.), *The Philosophical Works of Descartes* (Vol. 1), Cambridge: Cambridge University Press, 101.

Escobar, J. I., Swartz, M., Rubio-Stipec, M., & Manu, P. (1991) Medically unexplained symptoms: Distribution, risk factors, and comorbidity, in Lawrence J. Kirmayer & James M. Robbins (Eds.), *Current Concepts of Somatization: Research and Clinical Perspectives*. Washington, DC: American Psychiatric Press, Inc., 63–78.

Fauman, M. A. (1994) *Study Guide to DSM-IV*. Washington, DC: American Psychiatric Press.

Fowler, J. W. & Keen, S. (1985) *Life-Maps: Conversations on the Journey of Faith*. Waco, TX: Word, Inc.

Frank, J. (1961) *Persuasion and Healing*. Baltimore: The Johns Hopkins University Press.

Friedman, E. S., Thase, M. E., & Wright, J. H. (2003) Cognitive and behavioral therapies, in Allan Tasman, Jerald Kay, & A. Jeffrey Lieberman (Eds.), *Psychiatry: Therapeutics*, 2nd ed. Chichester, England: John Wiley & Sons, Ltd.

Frost, R. (1967) The road not taken, in *The Complete Poems of Robert Frost*, New York: Holt, Rineheart, & Winston, 105.

Hawton, K., Salkovskis, P. M., Kirk, J., & Clark, D. M. (1989) *Cognitive Behavior Therapy for Psychiatric Problems: A Practical Guide*. Oxford: Oxford University Press.

Hegel, G. W. F. (1952) *Hegel's Phenomenology of Spirit*, A. V. Miller (Trans.). Oxford: Oxford University Press.

Hollander, E. (1993) *Obsessive-Compulsive Disorders*. Washington, DC: American Psychiatric Press.

Houts, A. C. (2003) Discovery, invention, and the expansion of the modern *Diagnostic and Statistical Manuals of Mental Disorders*, in L. Beutler & F. Malik (Eds.), *Redefining the DSM: A Psychological Perspective*. Washington, DC: American Psychological Association, 17–65.

Joiner, T. E. & Schmidt, N. B. (2003) Taxometrics can "do diagnostics right" (and it isn't quite as hard as you think), in L. Beutler & F. Malik (Eds.), *Redefining the DSM: A Psychological Perspective*. Washington, DC: American Psychological Association, 107–21.

Jung, C. G. (1971) Psychological Types, in R. F. C. Hull (revision of H. G. Baynes, trans.) *The Collected Works of C. G. Jung*. Princeton, NJ: Princeton University Press.

Kellner, R. (1991) *Psychosomatic Syndromes and Somatic Symptoms*. Washington, DC: American Psychiatric Press.

Leary, T. (1957) *The Interpersonal Diagnosis of Personality*. New York: The Ronald Press Co.

Levi, A. F. (1959) *Philosophy and the Modern World*. Bloomington: Indiana University Press.

Linehan, M. M. (1993a) *Cognitive-Behavioral Treatment of Borderline Personality Disorder*. New York: The Guilford Press.

Linehan, M. M. (1993b) *Skills Training Manual for Treating Borderline Personality Disorder*. New York: The Guilford Press.

Malik, M. L. & Beutler, L. E. (2003) The emergence of dissatisfaction with the *DSM*, in L. Beutler & F. Malik (Eds.), *Redefining the DSM: A Psychological Perspective*, Washington, DC: American Psychological Association, 3–16.

Marx, K. & Engels, F. (1970) *Selected Works* (Vol. III). New York: International.

Meichenbaum, D. (1977) *Cognitive-Behavior Modification: An Integrative Approach*. New York: Plenum Press.

Nathanson, D. L. (1996) About emotion, in Donald L. Nathanson (Ed.), *Knowing Feeling: Affect, Script, and Psychotherapy*. New York: W. W. Norton & Company, 3.

Neenan, M. & Dryden, M. (2004) *Cognitive Therapy: 100 Key Points and Techniques*.

Hove and New York: Brunner-Routledge.

Robbins, J. M. & Kirmayer, L. J. (1991) Cognitive and social factors in somatization, in Lawrence J. Kirmayer & James M. Robbins (Eds.), *Current Concepts of Somatization: Research and Clinical Perspectives*. Washington, DC: American Psychiatric Press, Inc., 107.

Rush, J. & Beck, A. T. (2000) Cognitive therapy, B. J. Saddock & V. A. Saddock (Eds.) *Comprehensive Textbook of Psychiatry*, 7th ed. Philadelphia: Lippincott Williams & Wilkins, 2167–178.

Saddock, B. J. & Saddock, V. A. (1989) Typical signs and symptoms of psychiatric illness, in Benjamin J. Saddock & Virginia A. Saddock (Eds.), *Comprehensive Textbook of Psychiatry*, 7th ed., Baltimore: Williams & Wilkins, 677–89.

Schatzberg, A., Cole, J. O., & Battista, C. (2007) *Manual of Clinical Psychopharmacology*. Washington, DC: American Psychiatric Press.

Schreurs, A. (2002) *Psychotherapy and Spirituality: Integrating the Spiritual Dimension Into Therapeutic Practice*. London: Jessica Kingsley Publishers.

Shakespeare, W. *The Tragedy of Hamlet: The Prince of Denmark*. Act III, Scene I. Project Gutenberg, Champagne, IL.

Shorter, E. (1997) *A History of Psychiatry: From the Era of the Asylum to the Age of Prozac*, New York: John Wiley & Sons, Inc.

Stahl, S. (1996) *Essential Psychopharmacology: Neuroscientific Basis and Clinical Applications*. Cambridge: Cambridge University Press.

Steckel, W. (1943) *The Interpretation of Dreams*. New York: Liveright.

Stein, M. (1983) *In Midlife: A Jungian Perspective*. Dallas: Spring Publications, Inc.

Strasser, F. & Strasser. A. (1997) *Existential Time-Limited Therapy: The Wheel of Existence*. New York: John Wiley & Sons.

Sullivan, H. S. (1954) *The Psychiatric Interview*. New York: W. W. Norton & Company.

Taerk, G. (1998) Psychotherapy of functional somatic syndromes, in Peter Manu (Ed.) *Functional Somatic Syndromes*. London: Cambridge University Press, 237–55.

Tillich, P. (1957) *Dynamics of Faith*. New York: Harper & Row, Publishers.

Tsuang, M. T. (2002) Schizotaxia and the prevention of schizophrenia, in J. E. Helzer & J. J. Hudziak (Eds.), *Defining Psychopathology in the 21st Century*, Washington, DC: American Psychiatric Publishing, Inc., 249–60.

Turk, D. C., Meichenbaum, D., & Genest, M. (1983) *Pain and Behavioral Medicine: A Cognitive-Behavioral Perspective*. New York: The Guilford Press.

Vaillant, G. E. (1993) *The Wisdom of the Ego*. Cambride, MA: Harvard University Press.

Van Deurzen, E. (1998) *Paradox and Passion in Psychotherapy: An Existential Approach to Therapy and Counseling*. New York: John Wiley & Sons.

Wolff, W. (1950) *Values and Personality: An Existential Psychology of Crisis*. New York: Grune & Stratton.

Yalom, I. (1980) *Existential Psychotherapy*. New York: Basic Books.

Yalom, I. (2002) *The Gift of Therapy*. New York: Harper Collins Publishers.

JOURNALS

Akiskal, H. S. (2004) The bipolar spectrum in psychiatric and general medical practice. *Primary Psychiatry* 11: 9, 30–35.

Allen, L. A., et al. (2002) Psychosocial treatments for multiple unexplained physical symptoms: A review of the literature. *Psychosomatic Medicine* 64: 939–50.

Allen, L. A. et al. (2001) Somatization: A delibitating syndrome in primary care. *Psychosomatics* 42: 63–67.

Alpay, F. B. & Turhan, N. O. (2001) Intermittent versus continuous sertraline therapy in the treatment of premenstrual dysphoric disorders. *International Journal of Fertility and Women's Medicine* 46:4, 228–31.

Aragona, M. et al. (2005) Randomized double-blind comparison of serotonergic (citalopram) versus noradrenergic (reboxetine) reuptake inhibitors in outpatients with somatoform, DSM-IV-TR pain disorder. *European Journal of Pain* 9:1, 33–8.

Bachiocco, V., Scesi, M., Morselli, A. M., & Carli, G. (1993) Individual pain history and familial pain tolerance models: Relationships to post-surgical pain. *The Clinical Journal of Pain* 9:4, 266–71.

Barsky, A. J. (1983) Overview: Hypochondriasis, bodily complaints, and somatic styles. *American Journal of Psychiatry* 140:3, 273–83.

Barsky, A. J., Wyshak, G., & Klerman, G. L. (1992) Psychiatric comorbidity in DSM-III-R hypochondriasis. *Archives of General Psychiatry* 49:2, 101–8.

Bass, C. & Murphy, M. (1995) Somatoform and personality disorders: Syndromal comorbidity and overlapping developmental pathways. *Journal of Psychosomatic Research* 39: 403–27.

Blaustein, J. P. & Tuber, S. B. (1998) Knowing the unspeakable: Somatization as an expression of disruptions in affective-relational functioning. *Bulletin of the Menninger Clinic* 62: 3, 351–66.

Bradley, L. A., Arnold, L. M., Glass, J. M., & Clauw, D. J. (2008) Understanding fibromyalgia and its related disorders. *Primary Care Companion, Journal of Clinical Psychiatry*, 10: 2, 133–44.

Brown, W. A. (2002). Are antidepressants as ineffective as they look? *Prevention and Treatment* 5: Article 25.

Brown, W. A. (1998) The placebo effect, *Scientific American* 278:1, 90–96.

Brown, W. A., Johnson, M. F., & Chen, Mon-Gy. (1992) Clinical features of depressed patients who do and do not improve with placebo. *Psychiatry Research* 41:203–14.

Carlat, D. J. (1998) The psychiatric review of symptoms: A screening tool for family physicians. *The American Family Physician* 58:7, 1668–671.

Chand, P. K., Anand, S., & Murthy, P. (2000) A case of monosymptomatic hypochondriacal psychosis treated with olanzapine. *Annals of Clinical Psychiatry* 12:4, 247–49.

Cloninger, C. R., Reich, T., & Guze, G. B. (1975) A multifactorial model of disease transmission: Familial relationships between sociopaths and hysteria. *British Journal of Psychiatry* 127:23–32.

(No author specified) (2004) Depression and physical symptoms: The mind-body connection. *Journal of Clinical Psychiatry* 65:6, 867–76.

Creed, F. (2008) The relationship between somatization and outcome in patients with severe irritable bowel syndrome. *Journal of Psychosomatic Research* 64:6, 613–20.

Croom, K. F., Perry, C. M., & Plosker, G. L. (2009) Mirtazapine: A review of its use in major depression and other psychiatric disorders. *CNS Drugs* 23:5, 427–52.

Denninger, J. W. et al. (2006) Somatic symptoms in outpatients with major depressive disorder treated with fluoxetine. *Psychosomatics* 47:4, 348–52.

de Wied, M. & Verbaten, D. M. (2001) Affective pictures processing, attention, and pain tolerance. *Pain* 90:1–2, 163–72.

(No author specified) (2002) Dialectical behavior therapy. *Harvard Mental Health Letter*. 19:2, 1–3.

Doraiswamy, P. M. (2006) A randomized controlled trial of paroxetine for noncardiac chest pain. *Psychopharmacology Bulletin* 29:1, 15–24.

Edwards, R. R., Doleys, D. M., Fillingim, R. B., & Lowery, D. (2001) Ethnic differences in pain tolerance: Clinical implications in a chronic pain population. *Psychosomatic Medicine* 63:2, 316–23.

Evans, K. et al. (1999) Manual-assisted cognitive-behavioral therapy (MCAT): A randomized controlled trial of a brief intervention with bibliotherapy in the treatment of recurrent deliberate self-harm. *Psychological Medicine* 29:1–25.

Fallon, B. A. et al. (2008) A double-masked, placebo-controlled study of fluoxetine for hypochondriasis. *Journal of Clinical Psychopharmacology* 28:6, 638–45.

Fawcett, R. G. (2002) Olanzapine for the treatment of monosymptomatic hypochondriacal psychosis. *Journal of Clinical Psychiatry* 63: 2, 169.

Fink, P. et al. (1999) Somatization in primary care: Prevalence, health care utilization, and general practitioner recognition. *Psychosomatics*, 40: 330–38.

Fishbain, D. A., Cutler, R. B., Rosomoff, H. L., & Rosomoff, R. S. (1998) Do antidepressants have an analgesic effect in psychogenic pain and somatoform pani disorder? A meta-analysis. *Psychosomatic Medicine* 60:4, 503–9.

Gabbard, G. O. (2000). A neurobiologically informed perspective on psychotherapy. *The British Journal of Psychiatry* 177:117–22.

Gabbard, G. O. (1996) A reconsideration of objectivity in the analyst. *International Journal of Psychoanalysis* 75:15–26.

Garcia-Campayo, J. & Sanz-Carillo, C. (2001) Gabapentin for the treatment of patients with somatization disorder. *Journal of Clinical Psychiatry* 62:6, 474.

Goldstein, D. J. et al. (2004) Effects of duloxetine on painful physical symptoms associated with depression. *Psychosomatics* 45: 17–28.

Greco, T., Eckert, G., & Kroenke, K. (2004) The outcome of physical symptoms with treatment of depression. *Journal of General Internal Medicine* 18:8, 813–18.

Grossenbacher, P. G. & Lovelace, C. T. (2001). Mechanisms of synesthesia: Cognitive and physiological constraints. *Trends in Cognitive Sciences* 5:1, 36–41.

Guthrie, E. (1991) Brief psychotherapy with patients with refractory irritable bowel syndrome. *British Journal of Psychotherapy* 8: 175–88.

Halpern, J. (2007) Empathy and patient-physician conflicts. *Journal of General Internal Medicine* 22:5, 606–700.

Hamlin, C., Hitchcock, M., Hoffmeister, J., & Owens, R. (1996) Predicting surgical outcome for pain relief and return to work. *Best Practice and Benchmarking in Healthcare* 5, 258–61.

Han, C. et al. (2008) Fluoxetine versus sertraline in the treatment of patients with undifferentiated somatoform disorder: A randomized, open-label, 12-week, parallel-group trial. *Progress in Neuropsychopharmacology and Biological Psychiatry* 32:2, 437–44.

Han, C. et al. (2008) Venlafaxine versus mirtazapine in the treatment of undifferentiated somatoform disorder: A 12-week prospective, open-label, randomized, parallel-group trial. *Clinical Drug Investigation* 28:4, 251–61.

Hand, M. (1999) Antidepressant treatment of patients with diffuse esophageal spasm: A psychosomatic approach. *Journal of Clinical Gastroenterology* 28:3, 228–32.

Harth, W. et al. (2007) Psychopharmacological treatment of dermatological patients—when simply talking does not help. *Journal der Deutschen Dermatologischen Gesellschaft* 5:12, 1101–6.

Henningsen, P. & Lowe, B. (2006) Depression, pain, and somatoform disorders. *Current Opinion in Psychiatry* 19:1, 19–24.

Hickie, I. B., Scott, E. M., & Davenport, T. A. (1998) Somatic distress: Developing more integrated concepts. *Current Opinion in Psychiatry* 11:2, 153–58.

Hiller, W., Fichter, M. M., & Rief, W. A. (2003) A controlled treatment study of somatoform disorders including analysis of healthcare utilization and cost-effectiveness. *Journal of Psychosomatic Research* 54:4, 369–80.

Hoss, D. & Segal, S. (1998) Scalp dysesthesia. *Archives of Dermatology* 134:3, 327–30.

Hurwitz, T. A. (2003) Somatization and Conversion Disorder. *Canadian Journal of Psychiatry* 49: 172–78.

Humberto, M. & Escobar, J. I. (2008) Unexplained physical symptoms: What's a psychiatrist to do? *Psychiatric Times* 25:9, Special Report.

Isaac, A. & Wise, T. (2003) A low frustration strategy for treating somatization. *Current Psychiatry* 2:8, 33–50.

Johansson, B. B. (2004) Brain plasticity in health and disease. *Keio Journal of Medicine* 53:4, 231–46.

Keeley, R., Smith, M., & Miller, J. (2000) Somatoform symptoms and treatment nonadherence in depressed family medicine outpatients. *Archives of Family Medicine* 9: 46–54.

Keshen, A. (2006) A new look at existential psychotherapy. *American Journal of Psychotherapy* 60:3, 285–92.

Kjernisted, K. D., Enns, M. W., & Lander, M. (2002) An open-label clinical trial of nefazodone in hypochondriasis. *Psychosomatics* 43:4, 290–94.

Kooiman, C. G. et al. (2003). Is alexithymia a risk factor for unexplained physical symptoms in general medical outpatients? *Psychosomatic Medicine* 65: 911–18.

Kopp, R. & Kivel, C. (1990) Traps and escapes: An Adlerian approach to understanding resistance and resolving impasses in psychotherapy. *Individual Psychology* 46:2, 139–47.

Kroenke, K. & Swindle, R. (2000) Cognitive-behavioral therapy for somatization and symptom syndromes: A critical review of controlled clinical trials. *Psychotherapy and Psychosomatics* 69:4, 205–15.

Leibbrand, R. & Hiller, W. (2000) Hypochondriasis and somatization: Two distinct aspects of somatoform disorders. *Journal of Clinical Psychology* 56: 1, 63–72.

Linehan, M. M. et al. (1999) Dialectical behavior therapy for patients with borderline personality disorder and drug dependence. *American Journal on Addictions* 8: 279–92.

Lipowski, Z. Somatization: The concept and its clinical application. *American Journal of Psychiatry* 145: 45, 358–68.

Looper, K. J. & Kirmayer, L. J. (2002) Behavioral medicine approaches to somatoform disorders. *Journal of Consulting and Clinical Psychology* 70:3, 810–27.

Lynch, D. J. et al. (2007) The patient-physician relationship and medical utilization. *The Primary Care Companion to the Journal of Clinical Psychiatry* 9:4, 266–70.

Lynch, T. R., Morse, J. Q., Mendelson, T., & Robins, C. J. (2003) Dialectical behavior therapy for depressed older adults: a randomized pilot study. *American Journal of Geriatric Psychiatry* 11:1, 33–45.

Martin, R. D. (1999) The somatoform conundrum: A question of nosological values. *General Hospital Psychiatry* 21: 177–86.

Marty, P. (1968) A major process of somatization: The progressive disorganization. *International Journal of Psychoanalysis* 49: 246–49.

Maurer, I., Volz, H. P., & Sauer, H. (1999) Gabapentin leads to remission of somatoform pain disorder with major depression. *Pharmacopsychiatry* 32:6, 255–57.

Mayberg, H. S. et al. (2002) The functional neuroanatomy of the placebo effect. *American Journal of Psychiatry* 159: 728–37.

Meichenbaum, D. (1993) Changing conceptions of cognitive behavior modification: Retrospect and prospect. *Journal of Consulting and Clinical Psychology* 61: 202–4.

Meichenbaum, D. (1976) Cognitive factors in biofeedback therapy. *Biofeedback and Self Regulation* 1:2, 201–16.

Meichenbaum, D. (1996) Stress inoculation training for coping with stressors. *The Clinical Psychologist* 49: 4–7.

Menza, M. et al. (2001) Treatment of somatization disorder with nefazodone: A prospective, open-label study. *Annals of Clinical Psychiatry* 13:3, 1040–297.

Mercan, S. et al. (2007) Atypical antipsychotic drugs in the treatment of delusional parasitosis. *International Journal of Psychiatry and Medicine* 47:1, 29–37.

Muller, J. E. et al. (2008) Escitalopram in the treatment of multisomatoform disorder: A double-blind, placebo controlled trial. *International Clinical Psychopharmacology* 23:1, 43–48.

Newmark, T. S. & Al-Samarrai, S. (2004) Hypochondriasis and ECT. *Psychosomatics*. 45:1, 90–91.

Noyes, R., Jr., Happel, R. I., Muller, B. A. et al. (1998) Fluvoxamine for somatoform disorders: An open trial. *General Hospital Psychiatry* 20:6, 339–44.

Ogden, T. H. (1994) The analytic third: Working with intersubjective clinical facts. *International Journal of Psychoanalysis* 75: 3–19.

Okugawa, G. (2002) Paroxetine for treatment of somatization disorder. *Journal of Neuropsychiatry and Clinical Neurosciences* 14: 464–65.

O'Malley, P. G. et al. (1999) Antidepressant therapy for unexplained symptoms and symptom syndromes. *Journal of Family Practice* 48:12, 980–90.

Ostow, M. (1968) The consequences of ambivalence. *Psychosomatics* Sept-Oct, 257–58.

Paquette, V. et al. (2003) "Change the mind and you change the brain": Effects of cognitive-behavior therapy on the neural correlates of spider phobia. *NeuroImage* 18. Article in Press, 1–9.

Peterson, C. (1987) To be or not to be: A study of ambivalence. *Journal of Analytical Psychology* 32: 79–92.

Phillips, K. A. (2002) A randomized, placebo-controlled trial of fluoxetine in body dysmorphic disorder. *Archives of General Psychiatry* 59:4, 381–88.

Pia, L. & Tamietto, M. (2006) Unawareness in schizophrenia: Neuropsychological and neuroanatomical findings. *Psychiatry and Clinical Neurosciences* 60:5, 531–37.

Porcelli, P. et al. (1992) Alexithymia as predictor of treatment outcome in patients with functional gastrointestinal disorders. *Journal of Psychosomatic Research* 36, 5: 417–24.

Price, J. S., Gardner, R., Jr., & Erickson, M. (2004) Can depression, anxiety, and somatization be understood as appeasement displays? *Journal of Affective Disorders* 79:1–3, 1–11.

Rasmussen, K. G. et al. (2004) Relationship between somatization and remission with ECT. *Psychiatry Research* 129:3, 293–95.

Renik, O. (1993) Analytic interaction: Conceptualizing technique in light of the analyst's irreducible subjectivity. *Psychoanalytic Quarterly* 62: 553–71.

Rief, W. (2007) Analyzing the problems managing patients with medically unexplained symptoms. *Journal of General Internal Medicine* 22:5, 704–6.

Rief, W. & Hiller, W. (1999) Toward empirically based criteria for the classification of somatoform disorders. *Journal of Psychosomatic Research* 46:6, 507–18.

Rodin, G. M. (1984) Somatization and the self: Psychotherapeutic issues. *American Journal of Psychotherapy* 38: 2, 257–63.

Roffman, J. (2005) Neuroimaging and the functional neuroanatomy of psychotherapy. *Psychological Medicine* 28:1–14.

Sansone, R. A. & Sansone, L. A. (2003) Borderline personality: Different symptoms in different treatment settings? *International Journal of Psychiatry in Clinical Practice* 7:3, 187–91.

Sayar, K., Barsky, A. J., & Gulec, H. (2005) Does somatosensory amplification decrease with antidepressant treatment? *The Academy of Psychosomatic Medicine* 46:340–44.

Schwartz, J., Stoessel, P., Baxter, L. et al. (1996) Systematic changes in cerebral glucose metabolic rate after successful behavior modification treatment of obsessive compulsive behavior. *Archives of General Psychiatry* 53:109–13.

Sharpe, M. & Carson, A. (2001) "Unexplained" somatic symptoms, functional syndromes, and somatization: Do we need a paradigm shift? *Annals of Internal Medicine* 134: 9, 926–31.

Singer, T. et al. (2004) Empathy for pain involves the affective but not sensory components of pain. *Science* 303: 1157–162.

Smith, G. G. et al. (2000) Consultation-liaison psychiatrist's management of somatoform disorders. *Psychosomatics* 41: 481–89.

Smith, W. L. (1967) A psychotherapeutic technique for resolving impasse resistance. *Psychotherapy: Theory, Research, & Practice* 4: 162–63.

Smith, W. L., Hamlin, C., & Jonassen, E. (1999) Somatization: An independent variable influencing surgical outcome for pain relief. *Oakleaf*, USN MSC.

Spielmans, G. I. (2008) Duloxetine does not relieve painful physical symptoms in depression: A meta-analysis. *Psychotherapy and Psychosomatics* 77:1, 12–16.

Staab, J. P, Ruckenstein, M. J., & Amsterdam, J. D. (2004) A prospective trial of sertraline for chronic subjective dizziness. *Laryngoscope* 114:9, 1637–641.

Stahl, S. M. (2004) Anticonvulsants and the relief of chronic pain: Pregabalin and gabapentin as $\alpha_w\delta$ ligands at voltage-gated calcium channels. *Journal of Clinical Psychiatry* 65:5, 596–97.

Stahl, S. (2000) Blue genes and the mechanism of action of antidepressants. *Journal of Clinical Psychiatry* 6l: 3, 164–65.

Stahl, S. M. (2002) The psychopharmacology of painful physical symptoms in depression. *Journal of Clinical Psychiatry* 63:5, 382–83.

Stuart, S. & Noyes, R. (1999) Attachment and interpersonal communication in somatization. *Psychosomatics* 40: 34–43.

Taylor, G. J., Parker, J. D., Bagby, R. M., & Acklin, M. W. (1997). Alexithymia and somatic complaints in psychiatric out-patients. *Comprehensive Psychiatry* 383: 160–65.

Telch, C. F., Agras, W. S., & Linehan, M. M. (2001) Dialectical behavior therapy for binge eating disorder. *Journal of Consulting and Clinical Psychology* 69:6, 1061–65.

(No author specified) (1985) Treatment outlines for the management of the somatoform disorders. The Quality Assurance Project. *Australian-New Zealand Journal of Psychiatry* 19:4, 397–407.

Tumlin, T. R. (2001). Treating chronic-pain patients in psychotherapy. *Journal of Clinical Psychology* 57:11, 1276–278.

Vender, M. I., Kasden, M. L., & Truppa, K. L. (1995) Upper extremity disorders: A literature review to determine work-relatedness. *The Journal of Hand Surgery* 20: 4, 534–41.

Volz, H. P. et al. (2002) St. John's wort extract (LI 160) in somatoform disorders: Results of a placebo-controlled trial. *Psychopharmacology (Berlin)* 164:3, 294–300.

Voon, V. & Lang, A. E. (2005) Antidepressant treatment outcomes of psychogenic movement disorder. *Journal of Clinical Psychiatry* 66:12, 1529–534.

Voznesenskaia, T. G. (1999) Prozac treatment of chronic tension headache. *Zhurnal Nevrologii i Psikhiatrii Imeni S.S. Korsakova* 99:1, 34–36.

Waddington, J. L, Scully, P. J., & O'Callaghan, E. (1997) The new antipsychotics and their potential for early intervention in schizophrenia. *Schizophrenia Research* 28:2–3, 207–22.

Webster, B. & Shook, S. (1994) The cost of compensable upper extremity cumulative trauma disorders. *Journal of Occupational Medicine* 36:7, 713–17.

Wienfried, R. & Barsky, A. J. (2005) Psychobiological perspectives on somatoform disorders. *Psychoneuroendocrinology* 30:10, 996–1002.

Wise, T. N. & Mann, L. S. (1995). The attribution of somatic symptoms in psychiatric outpatients. *Comprehensive Psychiatry* 36:6, 407–10.

Wiser, S. & Telch, C. F. (1999) DBT for binge-eating disorder. *Journal of Clinical Psychology* 55: 755–68.
Zorumski, C. F., Rubin, E. H., & Burke, W. J. (1988) Electroconvulsive therapy for the elderly: A review. *Hospital and Community Psychiatry* 39:6, 643–47.

INTERNET SOURCES

Albertson, B., Brehm, J. R., & Alvarez, M. Ambivalence as experienced conflict. January 1, 2004. http://cas.uchicago.edu/workshops/polpsych/ambivalence.pdf.
Hoyt, M. F. & Meichenbaum, D. (1994) A conversation with Donald Meichenbaum. http://www.behavior.net/column/meichenbaum.
Knowlton, L. (2001) PET scans compare effects of drug treatment and talk therapy. *Psychiatric Times* 18:7, http://psychiatrictimes.com/p010744.html.
Liggan, D. Y. & Kay, J. (2005) Some neurobiological aspects of psychotherapy: A review, in Taming the anxious mind: How psychotherapy and medications transform the brain, CME. Co-Chairs: Philip T. Ninan, MD; Michael R. Liebowitz, MD; Faculty: Boadie W. Dunlop, MD; Sarah A. Feigon, PhD; Reviewer: Daniel K. Winstead, MD, http://www.medscape.com.
Schuessler, G. (2003). Neurobiology and psychotherapy. Lecture given at the Congress in Innsbruck on "Neurobiology and Psychotherapy," http://www.vr.de /data/files/117219/schuessler.pdf, 1–24.

OTHER SOURCES

(No Author) (2003) *Dialectical Behavior Therapy Intenstive Training Course (Manual).* Seattle, WA: Behavioral Tech, LLC.
John Philip Smith, letter to author, 10 October 2004.
John 15:13 KJV.
Novel atypical antipsychotics in non-schizophrenic conditions. (2003) Presentation of PsychCME, Program for Continuing Medical Education, Duke University Medical Center.

Subject Index

Author Index

About the Authors

W. Lynn Smith, PhD, ABPN, was an Associate Clinical Professor of Anesthesiology at the University of Colorado Health Sciences Center and for more than forty years specialized in the diagnosis and treatment of somatizing syndromes. He founded and operated the first hospital-based neuropsychological laboratories in the United States, where he did considerable research in personality, chronic pain, and psychosomatics. He developed and patented the Paindex® Test and Somatic Displacement Analysis® empirical testing instruments. He received the Distinguished Leadership Award from the National Academy of Neuropsychology. Having authored numerous articles as well as eight edited volumes, *The Mind-Body Interface in Somatization: When Symptom Becomes Disease* is his ninth and final book.

Patrick W. Conway, MDiv, has more than thirty years' experience in the fields of pastoral ministry and counseling. He has practiced as a psychotherapist in hospital-based psychiatric settings and is certified in the delivery of Dialectical Behavior Therapy. A graduate of Southwestern Baptist Theological Seminary, he has done additional work in the fields of Early Church language and literature and religious studies. His research interests include somatization, psychopharmacology, and existential psychotherapy. Currently a third-year medical student at the University of New England College of Osteopathic Medicine, he anticipates a second career in psychiatry. *The Mind-Body Interface in Somatization: When Symptom Becomes Disease* is his first book. He is the author of "The Beggar's Blog," highlighting issues related to medicine, psychology, and creative writing.

Jonathan O. Cole, MD, ABPN, was a Professor of Psychiatry at Harvard Medical School and a senior consultant at McLean Psychiatric Hospital (Belmont, Massachusetts). For more than fifty years he was active in psychiatric education and clinical practice. He was involved in research on most currently available antidepressants and helped introduce clozapine in the United States. In 2003, he received the Distinguished Life Fellow Award from the American Psychiatric Association. A prolific author, he produced well over 300 journal articles, reports, and monographs. With Alan F. Schatzburg, MD, PhD, and Charles DeBattista, MD, he was the author of a *Manual of Clinical Psychopharmacology*, 6th ed. (2007). *The Mind-Body Interface in Somatization: When Symptom Becomes Disease* represents his long-standing interest in psychosomatic medicine.